COACHES GUIDE TO SPORT PHYSIOLOGY

A publication for the
American Coaching Effectiveness Program
Level 2 Sport Science Curriculum

Brian J. Sharkey, PhD
University of Montana

HUMAN KINETICS PUBLISHERS, INC.
Champaign, Illinois

to Nancy and Brian, who've come to understand . . .
It's not the trophy
but the race,
Not the quarry,
but the chase.

Library of Congress Cataloging-in-Publication Data

Sharkey, Brian J.
    Coaches guide to sport physiology.

    Bibliography: p.
    Includes index.
    1. Sports—Physiological aspects. 2. Physical
fitness. I. Title.
RC1235.S518 1986   612'.044   85-24704
ISBN 0-931250-38-2

Editor: Stephen C. Jefferies
Developmental Editor: Linda Anne Bump
Production Director: Ernie Noa
Copy Editor: Olga Murphy
Typesetter: Sandra Meier
Text Layout: Cyndy Barnes
Illustrator: Jerry Barrett
Cover Design and Layout: Jack W. Davis

ISBN: 0-931250-38-2

Printed in the United States of America

10 9 8 7 6 5 4 3 2 1

Human Kinetics Publishers, Inc.
Box 5076, Champaign, IL 61820

ACEP Level 2 Sport Science Courses

ACEP Level 2 sport science courses are available to accompany the following texts:

 Coaches Guide to Sport Law by Gary Nygaard and Thomas H. Boone. The authors explain a coach's legal responsibilities in easy to understand terms and give practical advice for improving standards of care and safety for athletes.

 Coaches Guide to Time Management by Charles Kozoll. This innovative text shows coaches how to improve their self-organization and how to avoid the harmful effects of stress by controlling the pressures inherent in many coaching programs.

 Coaches Guide to Sport Physiology by Brian Sharkey leads coaches step-by-step through the development of fitness-training programs suitable for their sport and for the athletes they coach.

 Coaches Guide to Sport Injuries gives coaches information on injury prevention and on the immediate treatment and follow-up care for common athletic injuries.

 Coaches Guide to Teaching Sport Skills uses practical coaching examples to take coaches through the teaching/learning process and offers coaches valuable advice for improving their teaching effectiveness.

 Coaches Guide to Sport Psychology by Rainer Martens presents information on motivation, communication, stress management, the use of mental imagery, and other fascinating topics for enhancing coach-athlete relationships and for stimulating improved sport performances.

Each course consists of a *Coaches Guide*, a *Study Guide*, and a *Workbook*. ACEP certification is awarded for successful course completion. For more information about these courses, write to:

ACEP Level 2
Box 5076
Champaign, IL 61820
(217)351-5076

Contents

Introduction

I've been involved in sport for as long as I can remember. My first competitive experience was in a grade school boxing program. In junior high it was soccer, basketball, and baseball. High school brought football and track into my life, and in college I kept busy with swimming, track, and tennis. Then I retired, right? Wrong. I became a coach.

My first coaching position made me realize how much I didn't know about sport physiology and training. I began to read everything I could find on the subject, but I never found enough. In those days the field of sport physiology was just developing. Fortunately, as more scientists undertook its study and as more perceptive coaches added their observations, principles of training began to emerge. Today, dozens of journals communicate the science of training, and organizations such as the American College of Sports Medicine foster regular scientific meetings and symposia.

My personal love affair with sport continues—as a performer, fan, and sport scientist. I enjoy training and competition as much today as I did 20 or 30 years ago and still compete in running, cross-country skiing, and tennis. I enjoy the way training for one sport keeps me fit for another, how participation in sport adds excitement and purpose to daily activity. I hope I will never have to give up the challenge and satisfaction of competitive sport.

In the *Coaches Guide to Sport Physiology*, you will find the information you need to develop your own training programs. Questions such as why things work the way they do and why a specific exercise elicits a certain response are answered, and practical advice is given for improving the effectiveness of your athletes' training programs.

The book consists of five parts. Each part builds on the information given previously, and all of the parts, collectively, lead you through the process of developing sound training programs for your athletes. Let's briefly examine each of these five areas.

SPORT PHYSIOLOGY AND THE ATHLETE

In this first section you will learn how an understanding of sport physiology can enhance your coaching effectiveness. In this book the different physical qualities that contribute to an athlete's fitness for a sport are conceptualized into two distinct fitness components: muscular fitness and energy fitness. Most coaches find this distinction useful when organizing training programs for their athletes, for each component demands a distinctly different type of training. However, it is worth emphasizing that an athlete's total fitness for a sport depends on the effective combination of both fitness components.

When organizing a training program it is essential to understand and to apply the principles that govern the development of fitness. Those of you who have been through the American Coaching Effectiveness Program Level 1 course, or at least have read the Level 1 text *Coaching Young Athletes* will already be familiar with the principles of training. You are strongly urged to review key points of these principles that are presented in chapter 1.

If you have coached before, you will have noticed that individual athletes respond differently to the same training methods. Coaches need to understand why some athletes will not perform as well as others and consider individual differences when constructing and supervising their athletes' training. In chapter 2 we review the major reasons that account for the differences you observe between your athletes' responses to training.

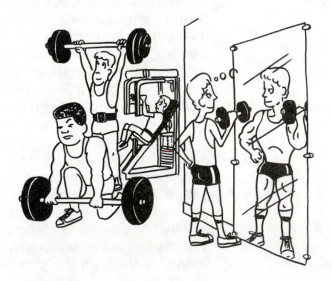

TRAINING FOR MUSCULAR FITNESS

Muscular fitness is the key to success in many sports. Football players need *strength* and *power*, distance athletes need *endurance*, sprinters need *speed*, and most athletes need *flexibility*, *balance*, and *agility*. Coaches need to know what elements of muscular fitness are important in their sport and how to develop these elements most effectively. The difficulty is in knowing how much strength, endurance, power, or one of the other muscular fitness components is needed for a particular athlete. You may know strength is needed in a sport, but how much is enough, and when should you switch to another form of training?

Muscular fitness training is the most widely misunderstood area in sport physiology. Only recently have coaches and physiologists begun the systematic application of science to the practice of training for muscular fitness. Previously, athletes trained for strength, regardless of the characteristics of their sport. They incorrectly lifted slowly in preparation for high-speed sports—and they neglected flexibility and muscle balance, thereby creating the conditions for musculoskeletal injuries.

Fortunately, the situation is improving. The experience of perceptive coaches, combined with laboratory and field observations and study, have led to the design of systematic programs and procedures for the development of muscular fitness. We are now better able to estimate how much strength is needed in specific muscles, to design more effective training programs, and to significantly increase an athlete's fitness level. We continue to learn how improvements in strength and endurance contribute to performance in sports.

In part 2, you will see how muscular fitness may contribute to success in your sport. Outlined in chapter 3 is some basic muscle physiology; then the physiological effects of training on each of the components of muscular fitness is examined in detail. In chapter 4 how to train for muscular fitness is explained, and appropriate training methods are described.

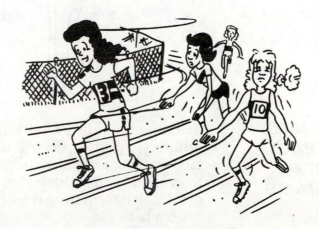

TRAINING FOR ENERGY FITNESS

The key to success in most sports is *energy production*— energy to run, jump, skate, wrestle, swim, or do almost every other kind of activity. We take energy into the body in the form of foods containing carbohydrate, fat, and protein. The energy stored in these foods is released by the muscle cells to power muscular contractions. The energy used for short, intense activities like the 100-m sprint is called *anaerobic*, which means without oxygen. The energy used to sustain prolonged activities, as in distance events, involves the metabolism of carbohydrate and fat together with oxygen, so it is called *aerobic*, which means with oxygen. Energy fitness training enhances the muscle's ability to utilize this energy, improves the heart and circulation, increases respiratory efficiency, and strengthens tendons, ligaments, and bones.

The focus of part 3 is on the energy sources and systems used in sport, showing how the energy systems can be improved through training. In chapter 5 you will learn how training enhances energy storage and production and will see the improvements produced by exercise in the respiratory and cardiovascular systems. Because the major effects of training occur within specific muscle fibers, coaches must remember to apply the principle of specificity when developing energy fitness training programs. Swimming is not a very effective training mode for runners, and long, slow running does little good for sprinters. Specific training methods for energy fitness are presented in chapter 6.

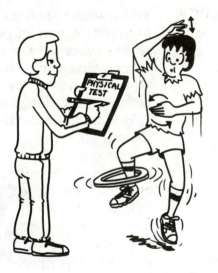

DESIGNING SEASONAL TRAINING PROGRAMS

Training must be individualized to meet the needs of each athlete. In part 4 you will learn how to develop individualized training programs. In chapter 7 is an explanation of how to evaluate your athletes' current fitness level using a series of tests that form the Athletic Performance Evaluation (APE). With a better idea of your athletes' current fitness level, you will be prepared to follow the advice given in chapter 8 for designing effective muscular and energy fitness training programs.

To help you understand the stages of training, I have included sample seasonal training programs for a wide range of sports, including those with low-, medium-, and high-muscular and energy fitness demands. These show how the various elements of training come together, how muscular and energy fitness fit into a year-round plan, how adjustments must be made to suit individual needs, and how the theory and principles of training can be applied to your sport.

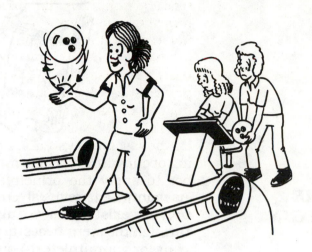

PERFORMANCE   Will a well-designed program for muscular and energy fitness prepare athletes for outstanding performance? Not completely. Performance is more than training; it is thoughtful preparation that includes good nutrition, adequate rest, and attention to other important details. Careful preparation is the key to consistent, high-quality performance.

Many athletes train long and hard to reach their goals, then blow it all with poor diet, lack of rest, or poor preparation. For example, Joanne had trained hard to reach the brink of national prominence as a distance runner. She had recorded one of the best marathon times for an American woman. But in her next race, a minor lapse in prerace preparation slowed her pace from a fine 2:36 to just finishing, painfully, in a veritable crawl. New shoes and a failure to lubricate her feet resulted in huge blisters, bloody feet, and several weeks of enforced inactivity.

Consistent performers prepare carefully, leaving little to chance. Less careful competitors are more likely to be inconsistent. Do not let your athletes squander months of hard work by neglecting preparation in the days and hours preceding competition. If you prepare for good performances, you are more likely to achieve them.

In part 5 you will be shown how to complete your training programs by attending to other essential details that affect peak performances. Setting realistic training goals, keeping accurate written records, learning how to peak for major competitions, avoiding the perils of overtraining, and controlling excessive stress will influence not only your athletes' success, but also the satisfaction you derive from coaching.

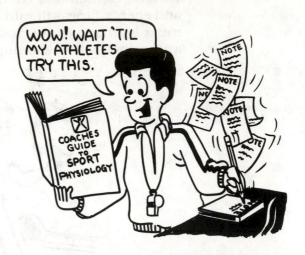

WHERE TO BEGIN

As mentioned previously, this book has been designed to build on your existing knowledge, and it is organized to lead you through the steps necessary to develop fitness programs relevant for your athletes. You may want to begin by first reading the table of contents and then by scanning the chapters to get a feeling for the material. As you get into the chapters use a highlighter or felt tip pen to underline important points. Keep a note pad handy to jot down ideas as they come to mind. As you read you will be challenged with exciting new ideas about muscle fibers and energy systems. I have tried to present the information as clearly as possible, but some new terms will appear. Most new words are explained in the text, or you can look them up in the glossary. In time, the terminology will become familiar and part of your coaching vocabulary. A *Sport Physiology Study Guide* is available from the American Coaching Effectiveness Program to help you apply this information to your own coaching program.

So get started and good luck! I hope this book contributes to your success and, more importantly, to your understanding and enjoyment of sport and coaching.

PART 1
Sport Physiology and the Athlete

Chapter 1
Introduction to Sport Physiology

Sport consists of preparation and performance—about 99% preparation and 1% performance. You need to make the most effective use of your preparation time so that your athletes can achieve high levels of performance. Chapter 1 begins with an explanation of sport physiology and training. Important principles of training are outlined, and muscular and energy fitness, the two key elements of the training program, are introduced. This chapter will help you understand how a knowledge of sport physiology can contribute to your athletes' success and to your understanding and enjoyment of sport and coaching.

SPORT PHYSIOLOGY

Physiology is the study of the body and how it functions. A physiologist studies the structure and operation of the tissues, organs, and systems of the body. Sport physiology is the study of the immediate and long-term effects of training and sport participation on the body's physical systems. Examples of immediate effects would include such changes as increases in heart rate, breathing, and body temperature. The long-term effects of exercise constitute training effects—the subject of this book.

Sport physiologists study training in several ways. One way is to observe how athletes differ from nonathletes: Are they stronger? Do they have more endurance? In what ways do they perform better? Another way is to examine how different training methods affect changes in strength, endurance, and other facets of performance. One of the best methods to measure training changes is to randomly assign athletes to training groups and to follow their progress. One group uses a new or varied experimental training technique, while the other group follows a traditional method or does not train at all. Using this research design, sport physiologists are able to conclude the physiological effects of a particular training method with more confidence.

Although it is always preferable to verify a training method, such as a new type of weight training or interval training with experimental proof, new techniques founded on unproven theories occasionally emerge. When this happens, sport physiologists look to the world of sport for validation. When experienced coaches and athletes use and endorse training methods and when those methods are physiologically sound, they can be included in the coach's repertoire.

TRAINING

Sport scientist Dr. Ned Frederick (1973) has described training as "a gentle pastime by which we can coax a slow continuous stream of adaptations out of the body" (p. 20). Training is a slow, subtle process; it cannot be rushed. Done properly, training leads to impressive changes in tissues and systems, changes that are associated with improved performance in sport. Rushing training or overtraining does not accelerate progress, but rather inhibits it.

PRINCIPLES OF TRAINING

Training is a systematic process. To train properly you must observe certain guidelines. You don't need to be an expert in physiology to conduct sound training programs, but you must understand and practice the principles of training. Those of you who have been through the American Coaching Effectiveness Program Level 1 course read about these principles in the ACEP Level 1 text *Coaching Young Athletes* (Martens, Christina, Harvey, & Sharkey, 1981). To refresh your memory and to inform those coaches unfamiliar with the principles of training, let's briefly review the key points of each principle.

Specificity Principle

Specificity is now viewed as one of the most important training principles to remember. This has not always been the case, however. In the past, athletes would run long distances regardless of the energy demands of their sport, the muscles involved, or even the type of sport itself. Research now clearly indicates that training should be specific for each sport. At least three different elements of specificity must be considered.

Specificity of energy systems implies that for sports requiring aerobic fitness, the athlete must follow an aerobic training program. Conversely, athletes in anaerobic sports should concentrate on anaerobic fitness. As examples, athletes in football, baseball, judo, and short running events must focus on short duration anaerobic training; excessive amounts of time spent on long-distance running are unlikely to enhance performance. A categorization of the predominant energy demands of most sports can be found on page 100. Further information on aerobic and anaerobic training is presented in chapters 5 and 6.

Specificity of mode of training implies that a maximal training effect is achieved when the mode of exercise is the same as that used during the skill performance. Quite simply, cyclists should pedal, swimmers should swim, and runners should run. Having your swimmers pursue a running program is less likely to improve their performance than organizing a similar workout in the pool.

Specificity of muscle groups and movement patterns emphasizes that using the correct training mode is not sufficient unless the same muscle groups used in the sport duplicate similar movement patterns. Every sport has its own unique muscular and movement characteristics. Can you remember trying a sport for the first time and waking up the next day stiff and sore? Perhaps you were surprised because you felt you were in good physical condition. Although you may have been fit for one sport, this experience illustrated the specificity of the fitness demanded by the new sport.

During training have your athletes model the identical movements demanded in their sport as clearly as possible. This must include a consideration not only of the movement pattern itself but also of the speed of movement. For example, if you want your athletes to run 5 minute miles, their training must be paced at a speed that will enable them to achieve this goal. Similarly, a weight program designed to strengthen the muscles used when hitting a baseball must include exercises that duplicate both the movement and speed of the swing. One of your most challenging tasks as a coach is to select appropriate exercises and, where necessary, to design your own to simulate the specific fitness demands of your sport. This is especially critical if you coach a sport that uses many "dryland" (simulation) activities because of seasonal variations or a lack of facilities (e.g., skiing, skating, ice hockey, and swimming). The steps for identifying the specific training demands of different sports are explained in chapter 8.

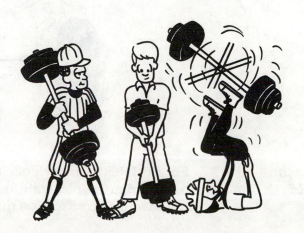

Overload Principle

Training must place a demand or overload on the body's system for improvement to occur. As the body adapts to the increased load, more load needs to be added. The training load can be controlled by adjusting the *frequency, intensity,* and/or *duration* of exercise. How to apply the principle of overload by varying exercise frequency, intensity, and duration is discussed in more detail in chapters 4 and 6.

Of all the training principles you must understand, the principles of *specificity* and *overload* are by far the most important to consider as you plan fitness programs for your athletes.

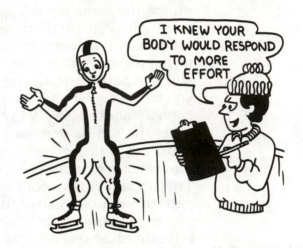

Adaptation Principle

Subtle changes take place in the body as it adapts to the added demands imposed by training. When training demands are progressively increased, athletes experience cardiorespiratory improvements, gains in muscular strength and endurance, and increasingly stronger bones, tendons, ligaments, and connective tissue.

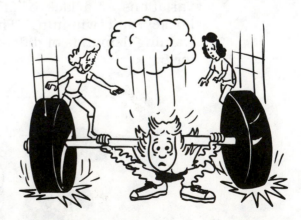

Progression Principle

For athletes to experience the adaptations stimulated by the overload principle, training must be progressive. If the training load is increased too quickly, the body is unable to adapt and breaks down. Careful control of the training load will ensure a steady rate of progression and will avoid the dangers of overtraining. Progression is a vital element to consider when designing a training program. As you follow through the step-by-step process of planning a training program in chapter 8, you will see how the need to ensure progression affects the selection of training exercises. Overtraining is discussed in chapter 9.

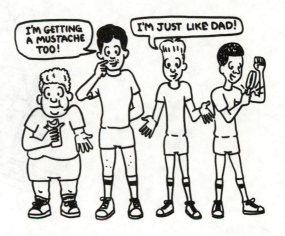

Individual Response Principle

Athletes respond differently to the same training. Heredity, maturity, diet, sleep, and other personal and environmental factors influence your athletes' abilities and attitudes toward training. It is unrealistic for coaches to expect all their athletes to respond similarly to the same training program. The many factors influencing an individual's response to training are discussed in chapter 2. Then in chapter 7 you are given a series of tests for evaluating the various physical qualities contributing to your athletes' fitness.

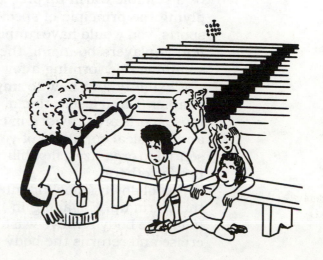

Variation Principle   Training programs must include variety to keep athletes interested and to avoid boredom. The concepts of *work/rest* and *hard/easy* are the basis of the variation principle. Training must always include periods of work followed by rest, and hard exercise followed by an easier workout. Coaches should vary their team's training routine and drills and also the training location.

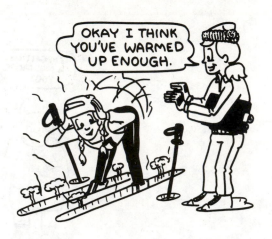

Warm-Up/ Cool-Down Principle   Every training session must include time to warm up and cool down. A warm-up preceding strenuous activity prepares the body for exercise and reduces the risk of injury. It has become traditional for athletes to begin the warm-up by performing a series of slow, stretching exercises, then to gradually move to more intense activities. Many coaches however, now prefer to have their athletes perform some easy-paced sport-specific activities *before* beginning to stretch. Explaining this, a former U.S Olympic track coach noted that he had more injuries during premeet stretching than during the track meets!

In practice this means that for your soccer players a drill involving passing the ball, conducted at an easy pace, may be a suitable warm-up preceding more intense practice. Applying the principle of specificity to the warm-up for other sports, you would have runners beginning with slow jogging, tennis players bouncing the ball and hitting easy strokes, swimmers performing a few slow laps, and so on.

Flexibility and how to improve it is discussed further in chapter 3, and a selection of flexibility exercises suitable for most sports are provided in chapter 4. Depending on the age and physical condition of your athletes, you may find it essential to organize a flexibility program for some athletes but not for others.

A cool-down following intense exercise is as important as the warm-up. Engaging in light activity (active cool-down) helps the body remove waste products generated during exercise and returns the body to its normal condition. A cool-down should include exercise of decreasing intensity, perhaps concluding with easy flexibility exercises.

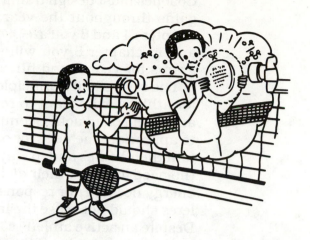

Long-Term Training Principle

Athletes experience long-term training effects by regularly and progressively overloading their body systems. Gradual improvements in physiological parameters contribute to enhanced performances. The principle of long-term training reminds coaches to be patient as they monitor the progress of their athletes and cautions them against pushing youngsters too hard, too fast, and too soon.

Research has shown that champion athletes typically train 8 to 10 years before reaching their performance peak. Daily and sometimes twice-daily training sessions may be necessary to achieve the highest performance standards. To sustain your athlete's interest in sport, you must organize developmental training programs that account for the athlete's age and experience. Young athletes pushed by overambitious and insensitive coaches not only quickly lose interest in sport, but they risk the harmful effects of overtraining.

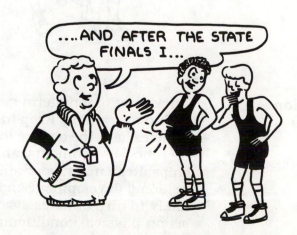

Reversibility Principle

Most of the adaptations stimulated by training are reversible. When athletes stop training, they gradually lose the physiological qualities that sustained their sport performances. Coaches must design training programs that maintain fitness gains throughout the year, especially in the off-season. In chapters 4 and 6 you are given advice for maintaining fitness, and in chapter 8 you will see how to develop training programs for year-round fitness.

The reversibility principle also has important implications for athletes who want to remain in good physical condition at the end of an active competitive career. Many athletes fail to appreciate the need for ongoing physical activity to maintain their bodies and to stay healthy. Especially important is the need to adjust their diet to correspond with their current energy needs. Your responsibility for the welfare of your athletes should not cease the instant your athletes stop playing. Despite an active athletic career, many athletes do not understand the principles of fitness and health. Advise them of the changes to expect during this transitional period and suggest practical measures to ensure their ongoing good health.

To these nine fitness principles, I would like to add one more—the principle of moderation. This is really a composite of key features from several other training principles but one worth stressing, especially to coaches of younger athletes.

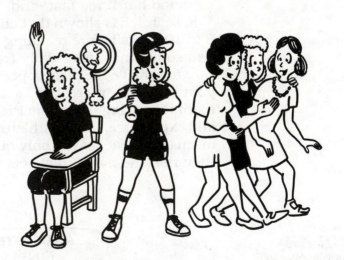

Moderation Principle

The secret to long-term success is moderation in all things, including training. Keep training in perspective. Be sure your athletes have the chance to meet family commitments, to fulfill school assignments, and to make time for social relationships. Remember, your athletes are seeking opportunities for personal development and for having fun. Nothing is more likely to turn athletes away from sport than an overemphasis on physical conditioning.

As your athletes become more skilled, you may need to impose training limits. Highly motivated athletes, seeing the benefits of training, often push themselves excessively and suffer harmful consequences as a result. Counsel your athletes to understand that while some training is beneficial, too much training can be counterproductive.

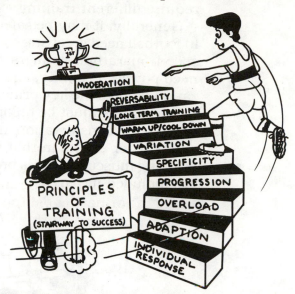

The principles of training will be repeated throughout this book, for these principles provide guidelines to help you develop your own scientifically based training programs. You will learn (a) how to design exercise programs to promote changes in the body and (b) how specific types of exercise will develop the fitness components needed for success in your sport. Throughout this book, I will discuss some of the physiological factors you should know to better understand your sport. Strength, power and speed, slow- and fast-twitch muscle fibers, aerobic and anaerobic energy systems, body fat and lean body weight are all concepts you will soon come to understand and will be able to apply to your program. First, let's consider muscular and energy fitness, the two key components of a scientifically based training program.

MUSCULAR AND ENERGY FITNESS

Sport-training programs are based on muscular and energy fitness demands. Knowing the demands of the sport helps you determine how much to train (intensity), how often to train (frequency), and how much time (duration) to spend to develop strength, endurance, power, and other fitness components.

Muscular Fitness

Muscular fitness consists of strength, muscular endurance, power, speed (including acceleration), flexibility, balance, and agility. Some events require considerable strength; others require muscular endurance, or power. Different sports and the various positions within each sport have specific muscular fitness needs. Thus, although two sports may require high levels of strength, because of differences in movement patterns, in muscle groups involved, and so forth, the sport-specific strength demands may be quite different and will require different training exercises.

Generally, it may be safe to assume that interior linemen in football need great strength, flankers and backs need more speed, marathon runners need endurance, and gymnasts need power, flexibility, and balance. However, this generalization ignores the key principle of training specificity: Training programs must be tailored to fit each individual in each sport with consideration made of variations between the positions or events in that sport. Recommendations for developing muscular fitness programs for the athletes you coach are included in part 2.

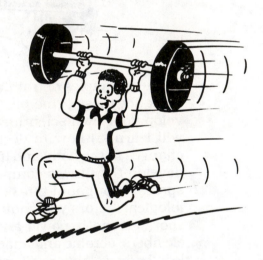

Energy Fitness

Energy fitness comprises the other half of a well-designed training program. Short-intense events that last only a few seconds, such as the shot put or the vault in gymnastics, require short-term (anaerobic) energy production. Longer events such as distance swimming or marathon running require more aerobic endurance, the ability to produce an adequate supply of energy throughout the event. Energy fitness training must be suited to the needs of the sport to achieve optimal results. In part 3 of the *Coaches Guide* various energy systems and how they can be developed are described.

Muscular and Energy Fitness Compared

These two components of fitness complement each other. Their distinction is only conceptual to help you better understand the training process. Just as muscles need energy to work, energy systems depend upon muscles to induce body movement. Similarly, when you train for muscular fitness, you will undoubtedly affect changes in the energy systems and vice versa. Other authors sometimes refer to energy fitness as cardiovascular fitness and may include a different definition of the factors that compose muscular fitness. Do not let this variability confuse you. All sport physiologists discuss the same physical qualities but have different preferences for presentation. I have found that most coaches like the muscular fitness/energy fitness distinction and find it a useful organizing model for developing their training programs.

SKILL TRAINING

Practicing game skills is often the most effective way of improving sport-specific muscular and energy fitness levels. Although skills and knowledge are useless unless athletes are fit enough to perform them, not all of your practice time can be spent on fitness training; nor will a general program of fitness development necessarily have the desired impact on sport-specific fitness needs. Teaching new skills and practicing known skills, learning offensive and defensive tactics, and understanding the rules and proper playing etiquette must be incorporated into the practice schedule in a way that also enhances sport-specific fitness.

How to combine muscular and energy fitness sessions with skill training is a challenging task for all coaches. You must look analytically at your sport, observe the specific movement patterns, identify specific fitness needs, then design activities that will train both skill and fitness. Your ability to perform these tasks will improve with experience and with sport-specific knowledge.

SUMMARY

1. To design effective, sound training programs coaches must understand basic sport physiology.

2. Sport physiology is the study of the immediate and long-term effects of exercise on the body.

3. Training is a systematic process that affects changes in the structure and function of the body's tissues and systems.

4. To conduct effective training sessions, coaches need to understand how the body responds to different types of exercise.

5. Coaches should observe the 10 principles of training when developing fitness programs.

6. The key elements of a scientifically founded training program are muscular and energy fitness. The unique physical demands of your sport will determine the

amount and type of muscular and energy fitness training that should be included in your coaching program.

7. Sport-specific skill practices are often the most effective way of combining skill training and fitness training.

Chapter 2
Individual Differences Among Athletes

Although most coaches work with teams, every team is composed of individual athletes. To apply the principle of individual response, you must show concern for the individuals you coach. Each individual will respond somewhat differently to the same training program. In this chapter, some of the reasons for these differing responses will be examined.

GENETIC INFLUENCES

Physical characteristics and qualities that are genetically inherited strongly influence an individual's response to training. Aerobic fitness—the ability to take in, transport, and utilize oxygen—is one such quality. A large proportion of aerobic fitness depends upon inherited characteristics such as heart size and muscle fiber type. Speed, acceleration, and power are also shaped by genetic factors. In spite of this genetic influence, all of these elements of fitness and athletic performance can be improved substantially with training.

Although relatively few individuals have the genetic potential to become elite international athletes, few athletes ever achieve their physical potential. In addition to their inherited physical advantages, the success of many champion athletes is also influenced by their determination to succeed. A challenging task for the coach is to help each athlete move closer to his or her physical potential. Sometimes this means you must reevaluate an athlete's suitability for an event, position, or even sport. Keep in mind, however, the level of achievement to which your athletes aspire. For example, a high school junior who is only 5 ft tall and who has parents less than 5 ft 6 in. will probably never make it in professional basketball, but that athlete might be capable of performing exceptionally well at the collegiate level. Similarly, although a youngster built for football will never make it as a champion gymnast, he or she might be capable of respectable and worthwhile gymnastic accomplishments.

Remember, too, that many champions have emerged after switching sports. An athlete may discover that a limiting quality in one sport can be a distinguishing quality in another. Helping your athletes achieve their potential should be a major criterion by which you evaluate your success as a coach.

During training, physical differences among athletes may make the same workout too easy for some athletes and too difficult for others. Coaches should try to recognize the differences in physical abilities among athletes and tailor their training programs to accommodate individual differences. Regardless of these fitness differences, always try to treat your athletes fairly. It is unrealistic to expect all athletes to perform at the same level when a workout is not individualized.

A key point to remember is how temporary athletic success can be, especially if you coach young people. In other words, the athlete who is currently the most successful in your squad may not ultimately be your most successful athlete. How many times have you heard or read about high school stars who failed to live up to expectations in college? Frequently, slower developers can eventually become leading performers. I once heard a coach compare this process with planting flowers in a garden. Each seed grows at a different pace: Some appear quickly then fade; others take time but eventually bloom to outshine all others. Take great care when trying to anticipate your athletes' potential for future success. Many capable youngsters are regularly rejected from sports because of an inaccurate evaluation of their sport ability.

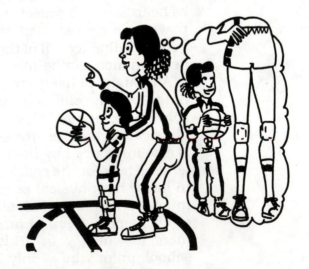

GROWTH, DEVELOPMENT, AND MATURATION

Young athletes grow, develop, and mature at different rates: That is, the increase in physical size and functional capacity of body systems is unique to each individual. Because attributes such as size, strength, and endurance are important factors in most sports, an athlete's growth and maturation rate directly influences his or her response to training and often his or her success in sport.

For example, during junior high school my friend Bob didn't have much success in basketball, his favorite sport, because he was too short. But over one summer he grew 5 inches. When he returned to school in the fall, the coach saw him in a different light (not to mention height). Bob now had the one missing factor he could not practice to improve—height. Bob eventually grew to 6 ft 8 in. and enjoyed an exciting basketball career in high school and in college. Thus, part of children's initial successes and failures in sport depends considerably on their level of growth, development, and maturation. Let's briefly consider the major stages of growth and development.

Early Childhood

The ages of 2 to 5 represent a period of rapid growth and development, especially in the nervous system, which is evident as toddlers gain better control of their developing muscles. This is the time to introduce fundamental movement skills such as running, jumping, throwing, catching, kicking, and striking. Children should experience the joy of movement and should be exposed to a variety of physical skills. These skills form the basis for more complex sport skills that will be learned throughout childhood and become fine-tuned during adolescence.

Most experts believe that early childhood is a crucial time for motor skill development. Children denied movement experiences during this stage may have difficulty acquiring complex skills later in life. Although some children are able to learn specific sports skills such as swimming or running before the age of 5, it is not advisable to push them at this stage. It is far more important that young, future athletes be provided many opportunities to explore and to enjoy a rich variety of movement experiences.

Late Childhood

The late childhood phase of growth and development begins at age 6 and continues to age 10 to 12. The emphasis should remain on teaching youngsters new skills and making sports fun. For most sports, this entire age group is too young to encourage specialization. Variety will help children grow and develop safely. In some sports, noticeably, gymnastics, figure skating, and swimming, the apparent reduction in the age of champion athletes has encouraged some coaches to consider earlier specialization. In addition to the health risks of excessive exercise, there is no evidence to support the assertion that increasing amounts of practice will necessarily produce better athletes. To sustain a child's interest in sport, all coaches are urged to focus on fun and variety and to avoid early specialization.

Early in this period, nerve fibers become completely insulated, which increases nerve impulse speed. More neural connections are made, too, resulting in greater muscular control and coordination. Fundamental motor skills learned earlier, as well as new, more complex sport skills, improve consistently when children are given ample time to practice them. During this developmental period, most of the body's systems show slow and steady growth; also, boys and girls are nearly identical in size and physical abilities.

Both muscular strength and endurance can be improved with training at this stage, but many child development specialists have argued that the improvements are generally small in comparision to the risks of injury and overtraining. In the past, the fear of injury prompted cautions against the use of weight training for preadolescent athletes. Now, however, the real danger is more closely related to inadequate instruction and supervision than it is to the use of weights. If youngsters are taught the correct lifting techniques and to avoid excessive loads, the risks of injury during weight training are probably no greater than when performing push-ups or similar calisthenic exercises. However, it is still too early for intensive fitness training. The optimal period for developing strength, endurance, and power begins a little later at the onset of puberty.

Repetitious practicing of fundamental game and sport skills will produce reasonable gains in strength and endurance during this preadolescent period. Prepubertal strength development may be accomplished with calisthenic exercises in which the body serves as resistance (e.g., chin-ups, push-ups, and dips). Endurance, power, and speed are best developed through play and team games that emphasize physical activity without eliminating fun. Repetitive skills practice also gives children a sense of mastery and increased confidence in their own physical abilities. Far greater strength and endurance gains can be achieved with less risk during adolescence, the next major growth stage.

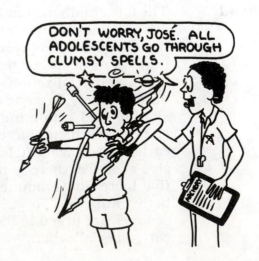

Adolescence

The onset of puberty marks the beginning of adolescence and typically occurs between ages 10 to 12 years in girls and 12 to 14 years in boys. Because boys' and girls' biological clocks are individually set for the onset of puberty, children of the same chronological age may be as much as 5 years apart in physiological maturity. More than any other stage, adolescence is a time of dramatic growth and maturation. Elevated levels of circulating hormones (especially testosterone for boys and progesterone for girls) promote dramatic changes in secondary sex characteristics, muscular development, and bone growth.

Performance differences, too, become evident between the sexes. In sports where physical size and strength are important factors for success, adolescent boys gain a performance advantage over their female counterparts. Females enter and finish the adolescent growth period approximately 2 years earlier than males. This additional 2 years of growth means that males are generally taller and stronger than females.

Minor difficulties in balance may occur during the peak period of growth for muscles and bones. This is because increases in strength lag behind muscle development, which, in turn, lags behind skeletal growth. With a mixture of exercise, rest, and adequate nutrition, this temporary situation fades, as do complaints of frequent fatigue.

Adolescent athletes who excel in practice and competitive performances are likely to be early maturers. Be careful not to discount the potential latent physical abilities of the more slowly maturing athletes. Often the slow maturers not only catch up, but surpass their early maturing contemporaries. The unique growth and maturational changes experienced by adolescents make them an interesting and challenging age group to coach.

Adolescent athletes often appear grown up, but they are neither physiologically nor psychologically mature. For example, the growth of long bones takes place at growth areas called epiphyseal plates located near the ends of the bones. These growth areas are less dense than fully calcified bone and thus are more susceptible to injury such as ligament detachment. Not until age 19 or 20, and sometimes even later, do the growth plates finish fusing with the bone shafts, thus marking the end of the adolescent stage of growth and development.

Training during adolescence produces relative improvements in strength and cardiovascular fitness that cannot be equaled later in life. Endurance training can increase oxygen uptake 33% or more. The heart muscle may increase in size, and well-planned strength training provides the stimulus for optimal development of muscles and power. Beginning at adolescence, the training load (determined by frequency, intensity, and duration) should be gradually increased as your athletes mature. Boys will usually gain more strength and muscle size than girls because of different levels of the growth stimulating hormone, testosterone. Despite this difference, strength training for girls can have a significant training effect. Flexibility deteriorates rapidly with age and may limit your athletes' future sport performances. Encourage your athletes to maintain and improve flexibility.

Despite the potential for physical development, too much training during a period of rapid growth and development can rob muscles and organs of the energy and nutrients they need to develop properly. Therefore, the coach and athlete must work together to plan a program of balanced work and rest and to ensure a healthy, nutritious diet. Shown in Table 2.1 are some general muscular and energy fitness training guidelines for children, adolescents, and adults.

You will notice from the chart how the intensity of training increases with age. This corresponds to the model of skill development shown in Figure 2.1. This model illustrates the typical developmental stages through which all athletes must pass to become elite performers. Athletes who achieve peak performances during adolescence are exceptions. Research has shown that the average age of Olympic champions has consistently remained in the mid-20s since the beginning of the modern Olympic Games.

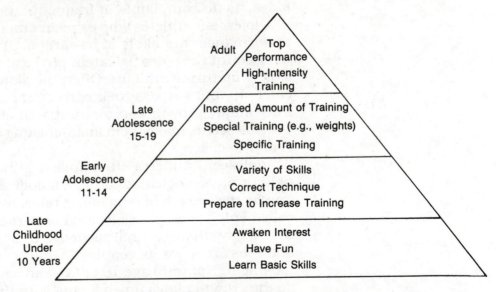

Figure 2.1. Age-based model of skill development.

The purpose and goals of training should change as children grow and develop. Athletes in some sports (e.g., swimming and gymnastics) seem to achieve top performances as young adults and then lost interest before they reach physiological maturity. Although in some sports this may be partly due to the financial basis of support, in general, top performances are achieved by mature, well-trained, well-rested athletes.

Table 2.1
Age-Based Training Guidelines

Growth Stages	Muscular Fitness Methods	Time	Energy Fitness Methods	Time
Children 6-10	Use body weight as resistance in general conditioning exercises (chin-ups, push-ups, etc.). Maintain flexibility.	15 min 3x/week	Team games with few playing restrictions. Emphasize involvement, play, and free expression. Avoid formal fitness-training methods.	Under 4 hr[a] /wk
Adolescent (early) 11-14	Use moderate resistance and more repetitions (over 10) on weight-training machines to develop endurance. Maintain flexibility.	30 min 3x/week	Continue to develop fitness through the use of team games. Improved aerobic ability is the main training goal. Introduce activities involving long, easy-paced intervals.	4-6 hr /wk
Adolescent (late) 15-19	Introduce high-resistance training (under 10 repetitions) and use of free weights to improve strength and develop power. Maintain flexibility.	45 min 3x/week	Increase training intensity. Mix long and short intervals. Train regularly at the anaerobic threshold.	6-8 hr /wk
Adult	Advanced muscular fitness training demands depend on specifics of sport specialization.	1 hr 6x/week	Prepare for peak competitive performances by developing a seasonal plan for energy fitness that integrates sport-specific requirements into the annual competitive cycle.	Over 8 hr /wk

[a]Usually 1-2 hr unless children are in organized programs (e.g., swimming) involving slow/easy distance training.

MALE AND FEMALE RESPONSES TO TRAINING

Males and females of all ages can benefit from muscular and energy fitness training. For prepubescent children it is unnecessary to separate children by sex for sport participation. During childhood, physical differences are often more apparent between individuals of the same sex than they are between sexes. Coaches working with this age group are encouraged to focus on individual development and to give children of both sexes equal opportunity to play on their teams.

During adolescence, although sex differences may affect patterns of sport participation, there is no reason why both sexes should not engage in strenuous fitness training. Research does not support any contention that vigorous physical activity can have a harmful influence on menstruation, future pregnancy, and childbirth. Only in collision sports, in which females are often at a weight and strength disadvantage, should female participation receive special concern. In many sports, skill, experience, and other matching factors influence performance far more significantly than do physical attributes.

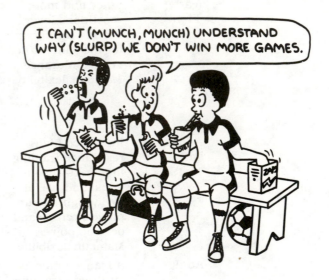

DIET AND NUTRITION

If your athletes do not eat an adequate diet and lack the essential protein, vitamins, and minerals they need to support growth and development, they will not be able to handle intense physical training.

The importance of diet and nutrition is well illustrated by the experience of Don, a friend of mine, who took a job as head basketball coach in an inner-city high school after finishing his master's degree. Don had never coached before; in fact, he had never even played basketball in college. Despite his inexperience, Don predicted he was going to turn his players into a powerhouse by teaching team defense. We were dubious, but he did it. How? Soon after he arrived on his new job he realized that his otherwise capable athletes were listless—low on energy. He discovered that few players ate breakfast, and that their typical lunch consisted of a bottle of soda pop and a chocolate cupcake. Don instituted a nutrition program, provided vitamins, and led his team to the runner-up spot in the highly competitive city league. The next year he won the league and was named coach of the year.

When you are coaching, remember that nutrition may be one of the reasons some of your players struggle to handle intense physical training. Proper nutrition and weight control is a vital part of fitness. For more information on this topic read the *Coaches Guide to Nutrition and Weight Control* (Eisenman & Johnson, 1982).

REST AND SLEEP

When I started teaching, I remember having some students wearily drag themselves into my 8:00 a.m. class. At first, I interpreted this personally as a sign that my class was boring; however, I have since changed my opinion. In some cases, I discovered that the students worked at night and were not getting enough sleep. Others were night people who just did not function well in the morning. (I must confess, though, that a few did find my class boring.)

Growing athletes need lots of rest, some more than others. Many of the changes that result from training occur during sleep; so explain to your athletes that those who miss sleep may lose these training benefits. Recommended guidelines for sleep for different age groups appear in Table 2.2.

Observe your athletes closely. If they appear overtired, insist they take time off and rest. Find out if they are getting enough rest and sleep. Do they have a job? Are they studying long hours? Are brothers and sisters keeping them awake? Try to find the reason for their fatigue and work toward a solution. If you look after your athletes' health and personal development, winning will take care of itself.

Table 2.2
Rest and Sleep Guidelines for Young Athletes

Stage	Hours Sleep[a]
Children (6-10)	10
Youth (11-14)	9-10
Young adult (15-19)	8-9
Adult	7-8

[a]Plus naps as needed.

LEVEL OF FITNESS

When your athletes are working in groups, have you ever noticed that some tire sooner than others? Your athletes' level of fitness depends on inherited physical characteristics and the extent of their previous sport experiences. Coaches should not be surprised to discover that a workout may be too easy for one athlete and too hard for another. Perceptive coaches quickly realize these differences and adjust the practice to account for individual differences.

One of the ways to account for individual differences is to measure your athletes' recovery heart rate (discussed in chapter 6). The recovery heart rate can tell you when your athletes are ready for the next training interval. Alternatively, you can group athletes according to fitness levels and give those with higher fitness levels a more intense workout. As your athletes' fitness improves, all aspects of the training program must be adjusted to ensure ongoing progress. For more fit athletes, the intensity, duration, and frequency of training should be increased. Try to avoid holding the more fit athletes back with those less fit, and do not force less fit athletes to go beyond their capabilities. By treating all your athletes as individuals, all will have a chance of reaching their potential.

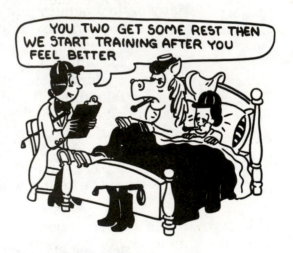

ENVIRONMEN-TAL FACTORS

Several years ago at a major eastern university, a young football player collapsed and died during practice. The athlete was performing poorly on a hot, muggy afternoon. Blaming his poor performance on laziness, the coach ordered the player to take several laps around the stadium track. Minutes later the young man dropped dead, a victim of heat stroke.

Individuals react differently to environmental stressors such as heat, cold, and altitude. Even some very strong athletes are unable to perform when the temperature or humidity climbs. If your team has to compete in a hot environment, encourage your players to drink lots of fluids, especially water. Dehydration robs water from the blood and cells and saps endurance. You should also be familiar with signs of heat illness, so you can keep a sharp eye on your athletes as they are working out.

ILLNESS OR INJURY

What should you do if athletes feel flat or listless? These feelings often signal the early stages of a cold or flu. The biggest enemies of young athletes in endurance sports are upper respiratory problems, including viral and bacterial infections, allergies, and asthma. Athletes who work too hard when they have a cold may make it worse. Instead of taking off a few days of training, they ruin weeks of past training by tearing down their bodies. Allergies have the effect of making athletes tired, which, in turn, increases the difficulty of practices or competition. Be sure you are aware if any of your athletes suffer from asthma or hay fever and if they are taking medication. These medicines tend to make the user drowsy and less energetic. Another danger, especially when coaching young athletes, is the tendency of youngsters to try to hide minor overuse injuries for fear of losing their place on the team. These injuries inevitably worsen, keeping the athlete out for weeks.

Bill Koch trained carefully for the 1982 World Cross-Country Ski Championships in Oslo, Norway. He planned his training to peak just before the February races. The first race of the championships, the 30 k (18.6 mi) proved his training was right on schedule. He won the bronze medal just seconds behind the winner. Days later, he became ill and was forced to drop out of a race. But Bill wasn't through for the season. His solid training base and time off from training provided him strength and recuperative powers. Bill recovered, skied the final races of the season, and became the first American ever to win the World Cup, the supreme title in cross-country skiing.

Only a fit and rested athlete could recover as quickly as Bill Koch. If you allow your athletes to run themselves down, minor colds and injuries can become major problems. Patience and understanding with sick or injured athletes will speed the recovery process and will enable them to successfully return to competition.

SUMMARY

1. Because individuals respond somewhat differently to the same training stimulus, coaches must be prepared to adjust training demands to suit each athlete.

2. Many factors that affect an athlete's response to training are inherited. Although these inherited factors place limits on an athlete's peak performance, few athletes ever achieve their physical potential. Coaches face the challenging task of helping their athletes approach this potential.

3. Athletes grow and develop at different rates; this influences their response to training and sport success.

4. Children aged 2 to 5 should experience the joy of movement and should be exposed to a variety of physical skills.

5. The emphasis on learning skills and having fun should continue into later childhood, ages 6 to 10. Specialization in one sport at this young age risks the child's health and ongoing interest in sport. Team games that include continuous activity and calisthenics are ideal methods of stimulating the development of muscular and energy fitness.

6. Adolescence is the most productive time for introducing specific muscular and energy fitness training methods; however, overtraining is to be avoided.

7. Prior to the beginning of adolescence, there is little justification on the basis of physical differences for organizing separate boys' and girls' activities.

8. Because of the growth differences between males and females that occur during adolescence, some separation of the sexes may be appropriate, depending on the nature of the sport. However, there is no evidence to suggest that either sex will not benefit from strenuous physical activity.

9. Athletes who fail to eat an adequate diet are less able to cope with the stress of fitness training.

10. Athletes who lack sufficient rest and sleep may lose the training benefits that occur during these periods.

11. The extent of an athlete's previous sport experiences, combined with inherited physical characteristics, will determine the fitness level an athlete may achieve. Coaches should try to account for differences in fitness levels by adjusting the intensity, duration, and frequency of training sessions.

12. The effects of heat, cold, and altitude can threaten the physical health of your athletes, in addition to limiting their performance potential.

13. Encourage sick or injured athletes to rest and allow sufficient time for complete recovery before they return to activity.

PART 2
Training for Muscular Fitness

Chapter 3
Muscular Fitness Components

A brief explanation of the structure and function of muscles is provided in this chapter. This information will help you better understand the underlying rationale for the training methods employed to improve muscular fitness. Then the effects of training on the separate components of muscular fitness will be examined.

MUSCLES

Muscles make movement possible. Muscle contractions move the skeleton so sport actions like running, swimming, jumping, and throwing can occur. Nervous signals originating in the brain are sent down the spinal cord to tell the muscles when to move. This process is represented in Figure 3.1. When performing new skills, it initially takes a conscious effort to contract a given muscle group, but with sufficient practice, the flow of nervous signals and the resulting contraction become almost automatic. Practicing a skill reinforces the nervous pathways between the nerves and muscles they contact.

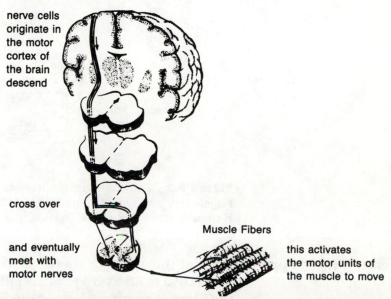

nerve cells originate in the motor cortex of the brain descend

cross over

and eventually meet with motor nerves

Muscle Fibers

this activates the motor units of the muscle to move

Figure 3.1. The control of muscles. Nerve cells located in the brain send impulses down the spinal cord to cause muscles to contract.

Muscle Fibers   Each muscle contains thousands of spaghetti-like muscle fibers (cells). Within the fibers are threadlike strands called myofibrils. These myofibrils contain protein components that enable the muscle fiber to contract and relax. Movement occurs when the proteins slide over each other and shorten the length of the fiber. Although it is still uncertain precisely how this movement occurs, one theory is that this sliding motion is made possible by the tiny cross bridges on one of the protein components. These cross bridges act like oars to pull one thread past another. The slight movement of each segment of a fiber collectively produces visible motion. Because the muscle fiber is attached to a bony lever, this converts the small contractions into large movements. Figure 3.2 is a diagram of the components of skeletal muscle from the muscle to the myofibrils where contraction takes place.

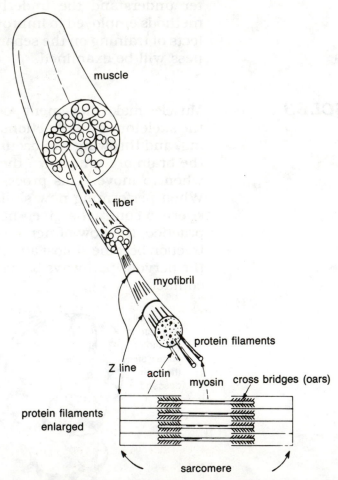

Figure 3.2. The anatomy of a muscle. Reprinted with permission from *Physiology and physical activity* (p. 20) by B. Sharkey, 1975, New York: Harper & Row Publishers, Inc. Copyright 1975 by Brian Sharkey.

Muscle Fiber Types   Each of the 1,000 or more slender nerves that enter a muscle activates an average of 150 muscle fibers. The nerve and the fibers it commands are called a motor unit. When the nervous system commands a motor unit to contract, all the fibers respond together. Motor units consisting of many muscle fibers will produce strong contractions, whereas motor units with only a few muscle fibers result in weak contractions. The response of a muscle depends on the number of muscle fibers in the motor unit and the number of motor units stimulated. This variability allows us the control that permits both fine, accurate movement and gross, large muscle movement.

All muscle motor units function in a similar fashion, but there is an important distinction between motor unit or fiber types. Two types of muscle fiber can be distinguished: *slow twitch* and *fast twitch*. Although most muscles have a mixture of slow- and fast-twitch muscle fibers, all the fibers in a motor unit are of the same fiber type. In Figure 3.3 you can see how slow- and fast-twitch muscle fibers mix together within the muscle.

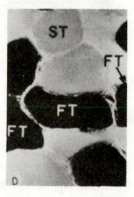

Figure 3.3. Slow- and fast-twitch muscle fibers intermingle in a cross section of human muscle.

For slower movements like walking or jogging, the nervous system recruits slow-twitch muscle fibers. For rapid or explosive contractions both slow- and fast-twitch muscle fibers are recruited. Fast-twitch fibers are fast contracting but are also quick to fatigue. Slow-twitch fibers contract more slowly, but they have more endurance. Some of the characteristics of slow- and fast-twitch fibers are shown in Table 3.1. You will notice two types of fast-twitch fibers: fast oxidative glycolytic fibers (FOG) and fast glycolytic fibers (FG). Fast oxidative glycolytic fibers share some of the characteristics of both slow- and fast-twitch muscle fibers: They are fast contracting but have moderate endurance.

As shown in Table 3.1, slow-twitch fibers are ideally suited for endurance work because of their high aerobic capacity (the ability to use oxygen). Fast-twitch fibers are more suited for short-term, intense anaerobic (nonoxidative) work. The fast oxidative glycolytic fibers, although suited for anaerobic work, can also be trained to improve performance in endurance sports.

Table 3.1
Characteristics of Muscle Fibers

Characteristics	Slow Twitch or Slow Oxidative (SO)[a]	Fast Twitch Fast Oxidative Glycolytic (FOG)[b]	Fast Glycolytic (FG)
Average fiber percentage	50%	35%	15%
Speed of contraction	Slow	Fast	Fast
Time to peak tension	.12 s	.08 s	.08 s
Force of contraction	Lower	High	High
Size	Smaller	Medium	Large
Fatigability	Fatigue resistant	Less resistant	Easily fatigued
Aerobic capacity	High	Medium	Low
Capillary density	High	High	Low
Anaerobic capacity	Low	Medium	High

[a]Oxidative means oxygen is used to produce energy.

[b]Glycolytic means glycogen is broken down to get energy for contractions.

Heredity Versus Training

While each of us may inherit a certain percentage of slow- and fast-twitch muscle fibers, the way the fibers are used (including the effect of training), also influences the percentage of each fiber type. Research indicates that elite distance athletes have up to 80% of their muscles composed of slow-twitch fibers, whereas sprinters and high jumpers have a higher proportion of fast-twitch fibers.

Training can influence fiber size. Strength training, for example, makes the fibers (especially the fast ones) larger in diameter. Training improves the performance of both fiber types, and some researchers believe that it may even be possible to change a slow fiber into a fast one, or vice versa. Recent studies suggest that with intense, long-term strength programs, the muscle fibers may split and form new fibers. This means the muscle could have more contractile units to apply force, and it may even develop new fibers. Consequently, the trained muscle becomes larger, or hypertrophies. Muscle fibers are capable of considerable adaptation when exposed to the stress of training.

COMPONENTS OF MUSCULAR FITNESS

Now that you have learned something about the structure of muscles, let's take a look at the following components of muscular fitness and see how they are influenced by training.

- Strength
- Endurance

- Power
- Speed
- Flexibility
- Balance
- Agility

Strength

What is strength? Strength is the maximum force that can be exerted in a single effort. All sports require a certain amount of strength, but strength becomes a priority in sports where heavy weights such as your body must be lifted, carried, or thrown. The strength of a muscle is related to its cross-sectional area or girth: The larger the muscle, the stronger it is. Strength training increases the contractile protein that gives the muscle its pulling power. As a coach, the challenge for you is to determine how much strength is required for specific skills and how to best train your athletes to develop and maintain the strength needed.

By comparing strength to performance, it is possible to determine if more strength is needed. If an athlete's performance improves with increased strength, then strength training is to be recommended. In long-distance endurance sports such as running, cycling, and cross-country skiing, only a certain amount of strength gain improves performance. In others such as weight lifting or football, athletes never seem to have enough strength. Athletes who have less strength with which to start will profit the most from strength training. Those who are already quite strong may see little improvement in performance because they already have sufficient strength for the demands of their sport. The exception to this occurs in events that are directly dependent on strength.

How can you tell when your athletes have enough strength and when they should shift to another phase of muscular fitness training? The characteristics of the sport provide us with some general guidelines. In continuous or longer duration events such as swimming or volleyball, athletes often have enough strength when the strength that must be exerted repetitively is less than 40% of the athlete's maximum strength, that is, when strength is at least 2.5 times the load. For short, intense events such as football and baseball, the strength required to perform the event should be less than 20% of the maximum strength in the muscle group, which means strength must be 5 times the load. Guidelines for determining whether your athletes have adequate strength are explained below.

1. Determine the typical load: Use a weight machine or pulley and have the athlete simulate the movement of a typical contraction required in the sport.

2. Determine maximal strength: Find out the amount an athlete can lift once (one repetition maximum, or 1 RM), performing the same movement tested in Step #1.

3. Comparison: If the athlete's maximum strength is not 2.5 times the load (5 times the load for short, intense efforts) the athlete may benefit from additional strength training.

To give you a better understanding, let's work through a practical example. Using a swim bench stroke simulator (modified from a weight-training machine), Tom, a swim coach, discovers that Alice, a 400-m freestyle specialist, exerts 20 lb of force in a typical arm stroke. This is the force exerted in a single arm pull during simulated swim movements.

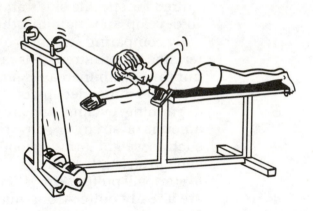

Her maximal strength doing the same movement is 40 lb. Distance swimming is an endurance event, so the coach uses the formula 2.5 × 20 and determines that Alice should have a maximum strength of 50 lb. The difference between this and Alice's actual strength suggests that she would probably benefit from strength training. This finding confirms Tom's feeling that a lack of strength is affecting Alice's technique and performance. With a little imagination and improvization, the movement of most sports can be simulated. However, if it is difficult or impossible to mimic sport movements and test for strength, coaches should look for other evidence of a strength deficiency. These include rapid fatigue, deterioration of skills, and loss of balance and accuracy.

Strength training will increase the contractile proteins of the muscle (actin and myosin) and toughen connective tissue. Some athletes will gain more strength than others because of their fiber type composition or hormone levels. The presence of the male sex hormone testosterone aids muscle development, thereby accounting for strength differences between males and females after puberty.

Eventually, all athletes hit a plateau that can only be raised by increasing the training load until at some point, further gains are not worth the extra effort. The demands of most sports are such that athletes will rarely approach their maximum strength potential. Strength peaks in the mid-20s for most people, although serious weight trainers have been able to increase strength beyond their 40th year.

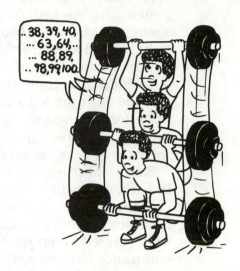

Muscular Endurance

Muscular endurance is the ability to lift a load repeatedly. Muscular endurance is usually measured by the number of repetitions an athlete can do with a certain weight or percentage of his or her maximum strength. Some sports involve repetitions with a fairly heavy load and require short-term endurance. Wrestlers, for example, have to overcome an opponent's body weight. Because the competition lasts only a few minutes, wrestlers need short-term endurance. Other sports (e.g., most cycling events) involve numerous repetitions with a light load, and this requires long-term endurance. In many sports, athletes will require both types of endurance to meet the changing playing conditions. For example, a cyclist who principally relies on long-term endurance for most of a race, needs short-term endurance when faced with a short, intense hill climb. At this moment, strength, together with the ability to produce and use energy rapidly, becomes critical.

Endurance training increases the muscles' ability to generate energy by enhancing the ability of the metabolic pathways to produce energy for contractions. Because short-term endurance training uses heavier resistance and fewer repetitions, it tends to increase strength and those enzymes used for short, intense efforts. Long-term endurance training, which applies the principle of lower resistance and more repetitions, improves the muscle's ability to utilize oxygen, thereby increasing endurance dramatically. Once again this demonstrates the principle of specificity—you get what you train for!

Athletes participating in sports or events that last a few minutes and involve a high resistance need short-term endurance. Longer events in sports, such as cycling, cross-country skiing, or running, demand long-term endurance training. Most sports require a combination of muscular fitness components. In basketball, for example, athletes must jump to shoot and rebound throughout the game. Because the load to be moved when performing these skills is the entire body weight, a combination of strength training, followed by short-term endurance training, will provide the strength to leap high and the endurance to keep doing it. When the effort is great but intermittent, short-term or intermediate endurance training applies. When the effort is continuous or nearly so, intermediate or long-term endurance training is required.

Every sport requires some muscular endurance training. In team sports like football or basketball, differences can decide the outcome of the game. Endurance is also important for athletes rehabilitating after an injury. Athletes should not be permitted to return to competition until both strength and endurance have returned to preinjury levels. Athletes who begin to participate in their sport before recovering muscular endurance risk the increased likelihood of reinjury when the muscles begin to fatigue.

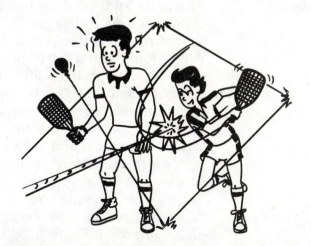

Power

Power is the rate of doing work. Power is an essential quality in many sports, for it represents the effective combination of strength and speed. This relationship is shown in the following formula:

$$Power = Strength \times Speed$$

Increases in strength or speed will increase power. And when power increases, more work can be done in less time.

Coaches generally think of power in big terms such as moving a 200-lb lineman out of the way in football, but power is useful in more subtle ways as well. Slightly more force (strength) or speed with each push-off allows runners to move with greater speed. A bit more speed with the racquet, bat, or golf club hits the ball faster and/or farther. In the past, coaches sought power by concentrating solely on size and strength, but today, coaches in all sports are emphasizing the effective combination of strength *and* speed.

Training can increase power in several ways—by increasing strength or speed and also by teaching athletes how to make more effective use of their available strength. The best power training seems to involve improving strength to an optimal level, then simulating movements specific to the sport, performed with resistance as fast as possible. More information about power training programs is presented in chapter 4.

Speed

Speed is related to the percentage of fast-twitch muscle fibers in the athlete's body. Because the quantity of fast-twitch muscle fibers is partially inherited, it is difficult to significantly improve an athlete's speed; however, it can be done. Speed of movement depends on the combination of two elements: *reaction time* and *movement time*. Reaction time is the time from the stimulus (e.g., the sound of a starter's pistol) to the beginning of the movement. Movement time is the time that elapses from the beginning of the movement to its completion.

Movement time is largely determined by fiber type and neuromuscular skill. (In a heavy resistance movement, such as the shot put, movement time will also be influenced by strength.) Although you may not change fiber type dramatically, you can improve your athletes' skill. Reaction time can be reduced with practice and by reducing the number of possible movement choices. For example, the quarterback reacts quicker and is more consistent when he has fewer options to consider. Improving speed is crucial for peak performances. A slight advantage in speed is the hallmark of the superior athlete.

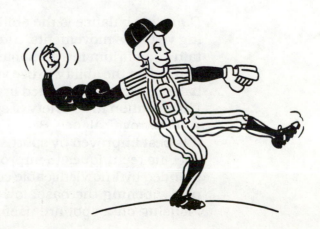

Flexibility

Flexibility is the range of motion through which the limbs are able to move. The natural range of motion of each joint in the body depends on the design of the tendons, ligaments, connective tissues, and muscles. Because many injuries occur when a limb or muscle is forced beyond its normal limits, flexibility training, which gradually increases a joint's range of motion, can help reduce the risk of injury. In addition to limiting an athlete's range of motion, tight muscles may impede optimum performance. Well-stretched muscles that flow easily through the range of motion require less energy and may facilitate better skill performance. Remember, however, that flexibility must be specific for the sport and for the individual. Some evidence suggests that extreme flexibility can actually destabilize joints or cause injuries. Unless you are coaching athletes in sports such as gymnastics, diving, or dancing, a moderate degree of flexibility is probably sufficient.

Improving flexibility, like the development of other fitness qualities, is a slow process. However, daily attention to flexibility relaxes muscles, stretches connective tissue, and improves the range of motion in joints. Flexibility exercises are usually included in the warm-up before vigorous exercise. Stretching prepares the muscles for work and can relieve muscle soreness, thereby making exercise more enjoyable. During and after a workout, stretching exercises are also recommended to keep the muscles and joints warmed up and ready to be put through their full range of motion. Stiffness and soreness often signal a need for more flexibility exercises.

Maintaining adequate flexibility is a year-round need and should be continued when your athletes eventually retire from sports. A lack of flexibility in the back and leg muscles, combined with weak abdominal muscles, leads to the all-too-common lower back problems, the scourge of millions of Americans. Back and hamstring stretching and abdominal exercises such as curl-ups should be part of everyone's daily fitness program. Be sure to teach your athletes the correct techniques for performing flexibility exercises. Many popular forms of these exercises increase the risk of injury and fail to produce the desired improvements.

Balance

Dynamic balance is the ability to maintain equilibrium during vigorous movements. *Static* balance is the ability to maintain equilibrium in a stationary position. Both types of balance depend on the ability to use visual information and input from balance receptors, located in the eyes, muscles, and inner ear. Participation in a variety of sport and movement experiences will improve balance. Because balance is largely task specific, it is best improved by sport-specific practice. In many sports, specific techniques to improve balance are routinely recommended by knowledgeable coaches. In gymnastics, for example, widening the base, lowering the center of gravity, and focusing on a spot are useful tips to improve balance.

Agility

Agility, the ability to change speed and direction rapidly with precision and without loss of balance, depends on strength, endurance, speed, balance, and skill. Practicing sport-specific movements will improve agility in that sport. Most coaches incorporate agility drills into early season practices. If agility is a problem for any of your athletes, have them participate in games and sports requiring rapid changes in direction such as racquetball, handball, and tennis during the off-season. Excess weight hinders agility and balance. If any of your athletes are overweight, suggest a sensible weight-loss program.

SUMMARY

1. Muscular contractions make all sports movements possible.

2. Muscles consist of thousands of fibers that are controlled by the central nervous system. Messages from the brain cause the fibers to contract, thereby resulting in movement.

3. There are two types of muscle fibers: Slow-twitch muscle fibers are suited for activities requiring endurance; fast-twitch muscle fibers contract more quickly (.08 and .12 seconds to peak tension for fast and slow fibers, respectively) and are suited for fast, intense activities not requiring as much endurance.

4. The proportion of slow- or fast-twitch muscle fibers in an athlete's body is influenced by heredity and training. Training will influence the size of the muscle fibers and can therefore affect performance.

5. Muscular fitness consists of strength, endurance, power, speed, flexibility, balance, and agility.

6. Strength is the maximal force that can be exerted in a single effort. The value of strength training can be estimated by determining whether your athletes' performances improve with increased strength.

7. Muscular endurance is the ability to lift a load repetitively. Different types of muscular endurance can be distinguished: long-term, intermediate, and short-term. The duration of your sport will determine the type of endurance your athletes need.

8. Power is the effective combination of strength and speed and can be increased by improving either or both of these two fitness qualities.

9. Speed is related to the percentage of fast-twitch muscle fibers in the athlete's body. Speed can be increased by decreasing reaction time and movement time.

10. Flexibility is the range of motion through which the limbs are able to move. Improved flexibility can reduce the risk of injuries and improve performance by increasing the joint's range of motion.

11. Dynamic balance is the ability to maintain equilibrium during vigorous movement. Static balance is the ability to maintain equilibrium while stationary. Both types of balance can be improved by sport-specific practice.

12. Agility is the ability to change speed and direction rapidly with precision and without the loss of balance. Agility is most effectively improved by practicing sport-specific movements.

13. The amount of training necessary to develop the components of muscular fitness depends on the requirements of the sport and on your athletes' existing fitness level.

14. Coaches should apply the principle of specificity when designing training programs and should endeavor to meet the sport-specific fitness needs of their individual athletes.

The purpose of this chapter was to review some of the theory upon which muscular fitness training methods are founded. In the next chapter specific training methods for developing the components of muscular fitness will be examined.

Chapter 4
Muscular Fitness Training

Training principles and methods for each major component of muscular fitness are presented in this chapter. You will learn how to evaluate your athletes' progress and how to maintain muscular fitness, and you will be able to see how muscular fitness quickly deteriorates when training stops. Once you understand the principles and methods of muscular fitness training, you will be ready to begin developing muscular fitness training programs for the athletes in your sport. This process is discussed further in chapter 8.

FLEXIBILITY

In this section the reasons for including flexibility exercises in muscular fitness training programs will be examined. Several methods for improving flexibility are also described. Specific flexibility exercises can be found in Appendix A.

Flexibility Training Principles

Flexibility exercises should be included in the warm-up that begins every muscular fitness training session. A few minutes of stretching before a vigorous workout can reduce the risk of injury and eliminate any leftover muscle soreness. Warm up with some light activity; then have your athletes concentrate on stretching the muscle groups used in their sport. Five to 10 selected stretching exercises are usually sufficient. One way to decide what needs attention is to have athletes stretch those muscles that are stiff and sore during or after practice. As a minimum, both you and your athletes should be sure to stretch the hamstrings and lower back to avoid low-back problems. Regularly remind your athletes of the importance of maintaining flexibility.

Flexibility Training Methods

Two recommended training methods are described, together with a method for developing flexibility with a partner.

Static Stretch

Static stretching involves slow movements to the point of stretch, holding the position for 5 to 10 seconds, and then relaxing. This technique is more effective than the old-fashioned bobbing method and is less likely to cause injury. If any athletes are suffering from muscle soreness, static stretching is a great way to bring relief. Have your athletes start on a rug or mat, stretching first the hamstrings and then the lower back. Then move on to other areas, using the contract-relax technique. Shown below is a static-stretching exercise for the hamstrings. Illustrations and descriptions of additional static-stretching exercises can be found in Appendix A.

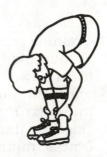

Bent knee stretch.

Contract-Relax Techniques

The contract-relax technique, a variation of the static stretch, helps muscles to relax and concentrates the stretch on the connective tissue, tendons, and joint capsules. After the usual static stretch, have athletes briefly contract a muscle (e.g., the calf muscle), then relax and do the static stretch again. Athletes should feel the stretch in the tendon after the muscle is relaxed. Work systematically around the body, contracting and relaxing the major muscle groups. Pictured below is an athlete using this technique to stretch the quadricep (thigh) muscles.

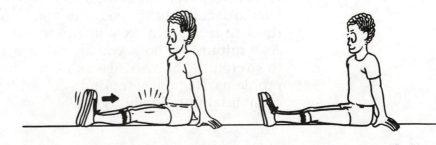

Contract-relax.

Two-Way Stretch

Certain stretching exercises are well-suited for partner work. For example, shoulder flexibility is enhanced when your partner *carefully* holds your arms from behind. But be careful: Warn your athletes that this is no time for horseplay.

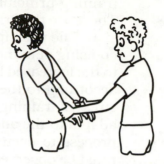

Shoulder stretch.

Maintaining Flexibility

It is wise to stretch daily, especially before an intense workout. Athletes without any muscle soreness can skip stretching on nontraining days. A moderate degree of flexibility can be maintained with one or two sessions per week, but high levels require more attention. Flexibility is lost rather slowly at first and is not hard to regain. However, it is wise to advise your athletes to maintain flexibility even during the off-season, for this makes the return to training less stressful.

STRENGTH

Strength Training Principles

Four of the 10 principles of training require special consideration when training for strength. These include specificity, overload, progression, and adaptation.

Training Specificity

The greatest strength gains will result from applying the principle of specificity. You may remember from the description in the Introduction to this book the importance of selecting training methods that simulate the movements required in your sport. Research indicates that performance improves more when the training is specific to the activity for which it is intended. Some years ago it was common for athletes to engage in "general conditioning programs" that developed overall strength or fitness. We now know that muscles important in the sport should be trained as specifically as possible. Conditioning programs should involve the muscles needed in the sport in ways specifically related to their use in the sport. The task of the coach is to design training programs that simulate the demands of competition.

Overload, Progression, and Adaptation

In addition to ensuring training specificity, three additional training principles relate directly to strength development: These are the principles of overload, adaptation, and progression. The principle of overload involves the imposition of increasing demands on the body systems. As the body adapts to the increased loading, more load must be added. The effect, according to the principle of adaptation, is that the regular stress of training produces changes in the body, and the body adapts to the added demands imposed by training. For this process to occur successfully, the principle of progression must be observed throughout the training process. Overload must be applied gradually, permitting the body time to adapt. If the load is increased too quickly, the body is unable to adapt and instead breaks down.

Applying these principles in practice is easy if you remember three key training variables: *intensity*, *duration*, and *frequency*. Intensity and duration are the two most important variables to consider to ensure overload is introduced progressively. It is essential to select a load that will stress the body but not cause it to break down. Based on research by DeLorme and Watkins in 1948, the concept of a *repetition maximum* (RM) evolved. A repetition maximum is the maximum load a muscle group can lift before exhaustion. If an athlete can lift a weight 10 times before exhaustion, this is referred to as 10 repetitions maximum (10 RM).

Research has indicated that optimal strength development occurs with between 6 and 10 repetitions, repeated at least 3 times with rest intervals between each set of repetitions. In the off-season, older athletes may benefit most from 5 to 8 sets or even more. Although there will be some variation between different sports, to develop strength effectively, athletes should repeat the strength training program at least 3 times each week. As a general rule, when an athlete can perform the maximum recommended number of repetitions with relative ease, you can increase the load. For exercises using the large muscles of the hips and legs, increases of 10 lb are appropriate. For other exercises, the weight should be increased in increments of 5 lb. These guidelines are illustrated in Table 4.1.

Strength Training Methods

Strength training methods are usually distinguished into three distinct categories: (a) *isometrics*, or static contractions; (b) *isotonics*, or weight training; and (c) *isokinetics*, or variable resistance. Each of these methods stimulates high-muscle tension, the key to strength development. However, differences do exist in the effect each training method has on sport

Table 4.1
Strength Training Guidelines[a]

Mode of Training	Repetitions	Sets[b]	Times/Week
Isotonic (weights)	6-10 RM[c]	3	3
Isokinetic (variable resistance)			
Slow (over 2 s)	8 FAP[d]	3	3
Fast (under 1 s)	15 FAP		
Calisthenics	6-10 RM	3	3

[a]Note: These are *general* guidelines. Later in this chapter and in chapter 8 some sample strength programs will be examined, and additional training variables will be considered.

[b]Sets—a group of repetitions. Athletes should do three sets for *each* muscle group.

[c]RM—maximum number of repetitions; the most that can be done with the weight.

[d]FAP—fast as possible.

performance. Let's consider some of the key features of each method.

Isometrics/Static Contractions

Isometrics are contractions against an immovable object such as a wall. In the 1960s isometric exercises were widely used by coaches and athletes in all sports. As our understanding of training has improved it has become clear that isometric contractions ignore a basic training principle—the principle of specificity. The use of static contractions is not suited for developing the type of strength necessary for performing dynamic sport movements. Static contractions are still valued only in sports that use static contractions (e.g., archery or shooting) or in rehabilitation programs when limbs cannot be moved.

Isotonics/Weight Training

Weight training involves the use of either weight machines or free weights and is the method preferred by serious weight lifters and body builders throughout the world. Typically, weight training exercises involve concentric muscle contractions: That is, the muscle shortens as the weight is lifted. However, it is also possible to exercise eccentrically by lowering a weight and allowing the muscle to lengthen. Interest in the use of eccentric contractions was stimulated by the observation that heavier loads and therefore greater resistance could be handled when lowering weights. Despite this difference, follow-up research has failed to report greater strength increases and indicates that eccentric contractions seem to produce excessive muscular soreness.

Isokinetics/Variable Resistance

Variable resistance training techniques represent the newest type of weight training. The principle of these techniques is to control speed and to vary resistance through a full range of movement. Specialized training equipment is required to use these techniques. Theoretically, isokinetic techniques appear to provide the most effective training methods for sports where strength and speed are important.

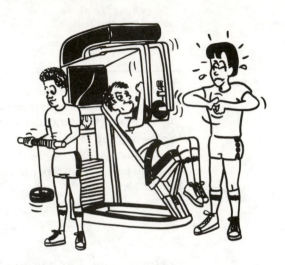

Weight Training or Variable Resistance?

Research has shown that weight training and variable resistance exercises seem to build strength equally well. However, for many sports, variable resistance contractions appear to offer the following advantages:

1. Variable resistance contractions provide high resistance and a training effect *throughout* the range of movement. When you lift weights, the contractions are hard at the start but easier as the exercise progresses and as the angle of contraction changes.

2. These devices are ideally suited for exercises to be performed as fast as possible. Many free-weight exercises cannot be performed at great speed without a risk of losing control of the weights. For these types of exercises, differences between the training effects of the two methods may significantly affect an athlete's sport performance.

3. Variable resistance training devices are able to work the muscles at contraction rates similar to those used during competition. This ensures the use of the same muscle fibers used in the actual performance. Ordinary weights or weight machines cannot duplicate this feature. As the sophistication of these training devices improves, it will become increasingly possible to simulate the specificity of different sport movements.

4. Variable resistance contractions do not usually produce muscle soreness. One cause of soreness is the

lowering of a weight (e.g., the letdown in an arm curl). If all you do is lift the weight, no soreness will develop. Many isokinetic devices eliminate the stress of lowering a weight.

Although variable resistance contractions appear to be advantageous for improving sport performance for several reasons, they are not without disadvantages. Currently, the high cost of many variable resistance devices limits their widespread availability. But perhaps more importantly, it's noticable that even the pro teams that can afford all types of training equipment are reverting to using free weights. An explanation for this is evident as you look ahead to the comparison of free weights and weight machines in Table 4.2. Free weights offer far more variety than any other training method. With weights, it's much easier to isolate and exercise sport-specific muscle groups. Another major advantage is the training effect on the important accessory muscles. Finally, the use of free weights trains *concentration*—a quality of tremendous value in sport, which is difficult to teach athletes by any other means. When athletes have to balance heavy weights, they must focus their undivided attention on the exercise. Few other occasions capture this degree of concentration.

Weight Machines or Free Weights?

Free weights provide the most inexpensive form of weight training. With the purchase of a bar and a selection of weights, every coach can institute a strength training program. The alternative to free weights is the weight machine. Although some machines boast variable resistance, rotary movement, or isokinetic features, most machines consist of an arrangement of weights and bars that facilitate isotonic training. The advantages and disadvantages of weight machines and free weights are compared in Table 4.2.

Table 4.2
Weight Machines and Free Weights Compared

Advantages	Disadvantages
Weight Machines	
Safe (self-spotting)	Limited number of exercises
No possibility of theft	Don't learn to balance weight
Save time	Don't train accessory muscles
Serve large numbers	Initial cost
Isolate muscle groups	Rotational movement is limited
Free Weights	
Greater variety of exercises available	Less safe than machines (require spotters)
Require balance	Greater possibility of theft
Train accessory muscles	More time-consuming (changing weights)
Isolate muscle groups	
Low initial cost	

Weight machines seem best suited for starter programs because they are safer to use and easier to control. However, as your athletes become more skilled, they need to learn how to use free weights to train the accessory or adjacent muscle fibers within a muscle group so that these are ready to assist when the primary fibers fatigue. When introducing weight training to athletes for the first time, you might consider using weight machines initially, then gradually teach the proper techniques for using free weights.

Organizing a Strength Training Program

Exercise Selection

Shown in Table 4.3 is a list of weight training and resistance exercises for different sports. These exercises are fully described and illustrated in Appendix B. Although suggested exercises are indicated for each sport, your final selection should be determined by seasonal priorities and the unique abilities of your athletes. When organizing a strength program, many coaches distinguish between the following four types of exercise: major, assistant, supplementary, and specialty.

Major exercises are those that have the greatest influence on strength development. The value of squats for leg strength and the bench press for upper body strength is evident from Table 4.3. In many programs these are considered the major exercises. *Assistant* exercises are those that have also been identified to have a significant training effect for a particular sport. Most programs include 1 to 2 majors and 1 to 2 assistants. *Supplementary* exercises consist of approximately 6 carefully selected but less vital exercises. The program is then completed by the addition of 1 to 3 *specialty* exercises, selected according to each athlete's individual needs. How to select and integrate exercises into a comprehensive seasonal training program will be explained in chapter 8.

Exercise Specificity

You are probably beginning to notice how the theme of specificity continues to be emphasized throughout this book. However, as you were reviewing the list of exercises in Table 4.3, did you think how a prescription of certain exercises for different sports seems to ignore this basic principle? A tennis coach could argue with some justification that an exercise like the bench press will not develop the specific strength that a tennis player needs. This is partly true; however, these exercises are still valuable for creating a foundation upon which greater training specificity can build. Also, depending on the abilities of your athletes and the contribution of mus-

Table 4.3

Recommended Weight Training and Resistance Exercises for Different Sports[a]

Exercises	Body Area	Aikido	Archery	Backstroke	Badminton	Baseball/Softball	Basketball	Bobsled	Boccie	Bowling	Boxing	Breaststroke	Butterfly	Canoeing	Cricket	Cycling	Discus, Shot Put	Distance Running	Diving	Equestrian
Arm curl	Upper and lower arm	✓			✓	✓	✓	✓		✓	✓			✓	✓	✓	✓			
Back extension	Lower back	✓	✓		✓	✓	✓	✓		✓	✓	✓	✓	✓	✓	✓	✓	✓	✓	
Bench press	Chest	✓	✓		✓	✓	✓	✓		✓	✓	✓	✓	✓	✓	✓	✓	✓	✓	
Bent-arm pullover	Chest	✓	✓		✓	✓	✓	✓		✓	✓	✓	✓	✓	✓	✓	✓		✓	
Bent-knee sit-ups	Abdomen	✓		✓	✓	✓	✓	✓	✓	✓	✓	✓	✓	✓	✓	✓	✓	✓	✓	
Bent-over rowing	Shoulder girdle	✓			✓	✓		✓		✓	✓			✓	✓			✓	✓	
Fingertip push-ups	Grip	✓			✓						✓								✓	
Heel (toe) raise	Lower leg		✓		✓	✓	✓	✓		✓	✓		✓		✓	✓	✓	✓	✓	
Incline press	Upper arm	✓	✓		✓	✓	✓	✓		✓	✓	✓	✓	✓	✓	✓	✓		✓	
Knee extension	Upper leg	✓	✓		✓	✓	✓	✓		✓	✓	✓		✓	✓	✓	✓	✓	✓	
Lateral arm raise	Shoulder	✓	✓		✓	✓		✓		✓	✓	✓	✓	✓	✓		✓		✓	
Leg curl	Upper legs	✓	✓		✓	✓	✓	✓		✓	✓	✓	✓	✓	✓	✓	✓	✓	✓	
Leg raise	Trunk	✓	✓		✓	✓	✓	✓		✓	✓	✓	✓	✓	✓		✓	✓	✓	
Military press	Shoulder, upper arms	✓	✓		✓	✓	✓	✓		✓	✓		✓	✓			✓	✓	✓	
Neck flexion and extension	Neck	✓			✓						✓									
Parallel bar dip	Shoulder, upper and lower arm	✓	✓		✓	✓	✓	✓		✓	✓	✓	✓	✓		✓	✓		✓	
Power clean	Trunk, shoulder girdle	✓	✓		✓	✓	✓	✓		✓	✓		✓	✓	✓		✓		✓	
Press behind neck	Shoulder		✓		✓	✓		✓		✓	✓	✓	✓	✓	✓		✓		✓	
Pulldown-lat machine	Shoulder girdle	✓	✓		✓	✓		✓		✓	✓	✓	✓	✓	✓		✓	✓	✓	
Reverse curl	Lower arm		✓		✓	✓		✓		✓	✓		✓	✓	✓		✓		✓	
Reverse wrist curl	Forearm				✓	✓				✓	✓		✓	✓	✓			✓	✓	✓
Shoulder shrug	Shoulder				✓	✓		✓		✓	✓		✓	✓	✓	✓	✓	✓	✓	
Squat (half)	Lower and upper back, upper legs	✓	✓		✓	✓	✓	✓		✓	✓	✓	✓	✓	✓	✓	✓	✓	✓	
Straight-arm pullover	Chest		✓		✓	✓		✓		✓	✓	✓	✓	✓	✓	✓	✓		✓	
Triceps extension	Shoulder, upper arm	✓	✓		✓	✓	✓	✓		✓	✓	✓	✓	✓	✓	✓	✓		✓	
Upright rowing	Shoulder	✓	✓		✓	✓	✓	✓		✓	✓	✓	✓	✓	✓	✓	✓		✓	✓
Wrist curl or wrist roller	Forearm	✓	✓		✓	✓	✓	✓		✓	✓	✓	✓	✓	✓	✓	✓		✓	✓

Table 4.3 (Cont.)

Exercises	Body Area	Fencing	Field Hockey	Figure Skating	Off/Def Linemen	Off Backs	Receivers	Def Backs	Kickers/Punters	Freestyle Swimming	Frisbee	Golf	Gymnastics	High Jump	Hurdling	Ice Hockey	Javelin	Judo	Karate
Arm curl	Upper and lower arm	✓	✓		✓	✓	✓	✓		✓	✓	✓	✓			✓	✓	✓	✓
Back extension	Lower back	✓	✓		✓	✓	✓	✓		✓	✓	✓	✓	✓	✓	✓	✓	✓	✓
Bench press	Chest	✓	✓	✓	✓	✓	✓	✓		✓	✓	✓	✓	✓	✓	✓	✓	✓	✓
Bent-arm pullover	Chest				✓	✓	✓	✓		✓	✓	✓	✓			✓	✓	✓	✓
Bent-knee sit-ups	Abdomen	✓	✓		✓	✓	✓	✓		✓	✓	✓	✓	✓	✓	✓	✓	✓	✓
Bent-over rowing	Shoulder girdle	✓			✓	✓	✓	✓		✓	✓	✓	✓			✓	✓	✓	✓
Fingertip push-ups	Grip																		
Heel (toe) raise	Lower leg	✓	✓		✓	✓	✓	✓		✓	✓	✓	✓	✓	✓	✓	✓	✓	✓
Incline press	Upper arm				✓	✓	✓	✓		✓	✓		✓				✓	✓	✓
Knee extension	Upper leg	✓	✓		✓	✓	✓	✓		✓	✓	✓	✓	✓	✓	✓	✓	✓	✓
Lateral arm raise	Shoulder	✓											✓						✓
Leg curl	Upper legs	✓	✓		✓	✓	✓	✓		✓	✓	✓	✓	✓	✓	✓	✓	✓	✓
Leg raise	Trunk	✓	✓	✓	✓	✓	✓	✓		✓	✓	✓	✓	✓	✓	✓	✓	✓	✓
Military press	Shoulder, upper arms				✓	✓	✓	✓		✓	✓		✓				✓	✓	✓
Neck flexion and extension	Neck	✓	✓		✓	✓	✓	✓					✓			✓		✓	✓
Parallel bar dip	Shoulder, upper and lower arm	✓	✓		✓	✓	✓	✓		✓	✓		✓	✓	✓	✓	✓	✓	✓
Power clean	Trunk, shoulder girdle	✓	✓		✓	✓	✓	✓			✓	✓	✓	✓	✓	✓	✓	✓	✓
Press behind neck	Shoulder				✓	✓	✓	✓		✓	✓		✓				✓	✓	
Pulldown-lat machine	Shoulder girdle	✓								✓	✓		✓				✓	✓	
Reverse curl	Lower arm	✓	✓		✓	✓	✓	✓		✓	✓		✓				✓	✓	
Reverse wrist curl	Forearm	✓	✓		✓	✓	✓	✓		✓	✓	✓	✓		✓	✓	✓	✓	✓
Shoulder shrug	Shoulder	✓	✓	✓	✓	✓	✓	✓		✓	✓		✓	✓	✓	✓	✓	✓	✓
Squat (half)	Lower and upper back, upper legs	✓	✓	✓	✓	✓	✓	✓		✓	✓	✓	✓	✓	✓	✓	✓	✓	✓
Straight-arm pullover	Chest	✓			✓	✓	✓	✓		✓	✓		✓				✓	✓	✓
Triceps extension	Shoulder, upper arm	✓	✓		✓	✓	✓	✓		✓	✓	✓	✓	✓	✓	✓	✓	✓	✓
Upright rowing	Shoulder				✓	✓	✓	✓		✓	✓		✓				✓	✓	✓
Wrist curl or wrist roller	Forearm	✓	✓		✓	✓	✓	✓		✓	✓	✓	✓		✓	✓	✓	✓	✓

Table 4.3 (Cont.)

Exercises	Body Area	Kayaking	Lacrosse	Long Jump	Luge	Motocross	Mountaineering	Orienteering	Pole Vault	Racquetball	Roller Skating	Rowing	Rugby	Sailing	Shooting	Skiing-Alpine	Skiing-Xcountry	Ski Jumping	Soccer	Speed Skating
Arm curl	Upper and lower arm	✓	✓	✓	✓	✓	✓	✓	✓	✓	✓	✓	✓	✓	✓			✓	✓	
Back extension	Lower back	✓	✓	✓	✓	✓	✓	✓	✓	✓	✓	✓	✓			✓	✓	✓	✓	✓
Bench press	Chest	✓	✓		✓	✓	✓	✓		✓	✓	✓	✓	✓		✓	✓	✓	✓	✓
Bent-arm pullover	Chest	✓	✓	✓	✓	✓	✓	✓		✓	✓	✓	✓			✓	✓	✓	✓	✓
Bent-knee sit-ups	Abdomen	✓	✓	✓	✓	✓	✓	✓	✓	✓		✓	✓	✓				✓	✓	
Bent-over rowing	Shoulder girdle	✓	✓	✓	✓	✓	✓	✓	✓		✓	✓	✓	✓	✓	✓	✓	✓	✓	
Fingertip push-ups	Grip	✓	✓											✓						
Heel (toe) raise	Lower leg	✓	✓	✓		✓	✓	✓	✓	✓	✓	✓	✓		✓	✓	✓	✓	✓	✓
Incline press	Upper arm	✓	✓			✓	✓					✓								
Knee extension	Upper leg	✓	✓	✓	✓	✓	✓	✓	✓	✓	✓	✓	✓	✓	✓	✓	✓		✓	✓
Lateral arm raise	Shoulder	✓																		
Leg curl	Upper legs	✓	✓	✓		✓	✓	✓	✓	✓	✓	✓	✓	✓	✓	✓	✓			
Leg raise	Trunk	✓	✓	✓	✓	✓	✓	✓			✓	✓	✓	✓						
Military press	Shoulder, upper arms	✓	✓			✓	✓	✓			✓	✓	✓	✓	✓	✓	✓	✓	✓	✓
Neck flexion and extension	Neck																			
Parallel bar dip	Shoulder, upper and lower arm	✓	✓	✓	✓	✓	✓	✓	✓	✓	✓	✓	✓	✓						✓
Power clean	Trunk, shoulder girdle	✓	✓	✓	✓	✓	✓			✓	✓	✓	✓		✓	✓	✓	✓		✓
Press behind neck	Shoulder	✓								✓										
Pulldown-lat machine	Shoulder girdle	✓	✓	✓	✓	✓	✓	✓	✓	✓	✓	✓	✓	✓		✓	✓			
Reverse curl	Lower arm	✓	✓		✓	✓	✓					✓	✓	✓	✓					
Reverse wrist curl	Forearm	✓	✓		✓	✓	✓				✓	✓			✓					
Shoulder shrug	Shoulder	✓	✓	✓	✓	✓	✓	✓	✓	✓	✓	✓	✓	✓	✓					
Squat (half)	Lower and upper back, upper legs	✓	✓	✓	✓	✓	✓	✓	✓	✓	✓	✓	✓	✓	✓	✓	✓	✓	✓	✓
Straight-arm pullover	Chest	✓	✓	✓	✓	✓	✓	✓		✓	✓	✓	✓	✓	✓	✓	✓	✓		✓
Triceps extension	Shoulder, upper arm	✓	✓	✓	✓	✓	✓				✓	✓	✓	✓	✓	✓		✓		
Upright rowing	Shoulder	✓	✓	✓	✓	✓	✓	✓	✓			✓	✓		✓	✓		✓		
Wrist curl or wrist roller	Forearm	✓	✓		✓	✓	✓				✓	✓	✓	✓	✓			✓		

Table 4.3 (Cont.)

Exercises	Body Area	Sprinting	Squash	Surfing	Synchronized Swimming	Table Tennis	Taekwondo	Team Handball	Tennis	Triple Jump	Volleyball	Water Polo	Weight Lifting	Wrestling
Arm curl	Upper and lower arm	✓	✓	✓	✓	✓	✓	✓	✓		✓	✓	✓	✓
Back extension	Lower back	✓	✓	✓	✓	✓	✓	✓	✓		✓	✓	✓	✓
Bench press	Chest	✓	✓	✓	✓	✓	✓	✓	✓		✓	✓	✓	✓
Bent-arm pullover	Chest	✓	✓	✓	✓		✓	✓	✓		✓	✓	✓	✓
Bent-knee sit-ups	Abdomen	✓	✓	✓	✓	✓	✓	✓	✓		✓	✓	✓	✓
Bent-over rowing	Shoulder girdle	✓	✓	✓	✓		✓	✓	✓		✓	✓	✓	✓
Fingertip push-ups	Grip		✓				✓	✓	✓			✓	✓	✓
Heel (toe) raise	Lower leg	✓	✓	✓		✓	✓	✓	✓		✓	✓	✓	✓
Incline press	Upper arm	✓	✓	✓	✓	✓	✓	✓	✓		✓	✓	✓	✓
Knee extension	Upper leg	✓	✓	✓		✓	✓	✓	✓		✓	✓	✓	✓
Lateral arm raise	Shoulder	✓	✓	✓		✓	✓	✓	✓		✓	✓	✓	✓
Leg curl	Upper legs	✓	✓	✓	✓	✓	✓	✓	✓		✓	✓	✓	✓
Leg raise	Trunk	✓	✓	✓	✓	✓	✓	✓	✓		✓	✓	✓	✓
Military press	Shoulder, upper arms	✓					✓	✓	✓		✓	✓	✓	✓
Neck flexion and extension	Neck													✓
Parallel bar dip	Shoulder, upper and lower arm		✓	✓	✓	✓	✓	✓	✓	✓	✓	✓	✓	✓
Power clean	Trunk, shoulder girdle	✓					✓	✓		✓		✓	✓	✓
Press behind neck	Shoulder		✓				✓	✓	✓		✓	✓	✓	✓
Pulldown-lat machine	Shoulder girdle	✓	✓				✓	✓	✓		✓	✓	✓	✓
Reverse curl	Lower arm		✓				✓	✓	✓		✓	✓	✓	✓
Reverse wrist curl	Forearm		✓				✓	✓	✓		✓	✓	✓	✓
Shoulder shrug	Shoulder		✓	✓			✓	✓	✓		✓	✓	✓	✓
Squat (half)	Lower and upper back, upper legs	✓	✓	✓		✓	✓	✓	✓	✓	✓	✓	✓	✓
Straight-arm pullover	Chest	✓	✓	✓	✓	✓	✓	✓	✓	✓	✓	✓	✓	✓
Triceps extension	Shoulder, upper arm	✓	✓	✓		✓	✓	✓	✓	✓	✓	✓	✓	✓
Upright rowing	Shoulder	✓					✓	✓	✓	✓	✓	✓	✓	✓
Wrist curl or wrist roller	Forearm	✓	✓				✓	✓	✓		✓	✓	✓	✓

ᵃ(Adapted from Fox, 1984.)

cular fitness to performance in your sport, this may be as specific as you care to view the training process.

For even greater benefits, you might like to consider how you could modify existing exercises or develop new training methods to more closely simulate sport-specific movements. With a little imagination you will probably find that the training principles for developing most or all of the components of muscular fitness can be applied to sport-specific skills. For example, a shot putter could use shots of varying weights: a heavier shot to develop strength and a softball to train for speed. To improve strength/endurance for poling in cross-country skiing, a lat machine can be used, or pulleys attached to weights could be set at different heights to exercise different patterns of the arm movement. By varying the resistance, the skier can determine the training effect. The introduction of sport-specific training methods becomes increasingly more beneficial as athletes enter the competitive season. Seasonal training will be discussed in more detail in chapter 8.

Exercise Order

As a general principle you should remember to select exercises that alternate the training effect between different muscle groups and permit adequate recovery. Successive exercises should not stress the same muscle groups. For example, leg curls and knee extensions should not follow one another because they both exercise the upper legs. Another consideration when arranging the order of exercises is to exercise the larger muscle groups (e.g., the legs) before the smaller groups (e.g., the wrist). This ensures that the larger muscle groups receive the correct overload.

In practice, some coaches modify this general principle and tell their athletes to complete *all* sets of major exercises before beginning on assistant exercises. Thus, an athlete might complete 3 to 5 sets of squats, then 3 to 5 sets of bench presses before progressing to the next part of the training program. Finally, remember to train opposite muscle groups to maintain a balance of strength on both sides of a joint (e.g., the thighs and hamstrings).

Starting to Exercise

To assess the starting point for a program, a little experimentation is necessary. The usual way to begin is to have your athletes perform each of the selected exercises and to adjust the loading of the bar until the athlete can perform *one* repetition only (one repetition maximum, or 1 RM). Before doing this, however, a word of caution is necessary. The risk of injury is greatest when your athletes attempt maximal contractions, especially when using free weights, for these stress body parts other than those being tested.

Whenever possible use machines to assess maximum lifts; these isolate the specific muscle groups to be tested. Remember, also, that the 1 RM is just an estimate to help you establish a starting point. It is unnecessary to push your athletes to their limit to make this estimate, and for young athletes this practice risks serious debilitating injuries.

Calculating
Starting Weights

Once you have estimated your athletes' 1 RM, a little more experimentation is necessary to find the load the athlete can lift to perform the number of repetitions (reps) in your program. Guidelines for calculating approximate starting weights based on 1 RM figures for the bench press are shown in the following chart. With experience you will be able to develop similar charts for each exercise included in your athletes' training program.

1 RM (lb)	Starting Weight (lb)
45-55	20
60-80	35
80-100	50
105-125	75
130-150	95
150-185	115
185+	135

Deciding the
Training Load

When you have established a starting weight, you must decide on the number of sets and reps for each exercise. The general guidelines given earlier in this chapter for optimal strength development were 3 sets of 6 to 10 reps. Most strength and conditioning coaches would view this as the minimum for effective strength development, especially in off-season or preseason programs for sports in which strength plays a vital role. For a sport like golf, 3 sets might be sufficient to meet an athlete's strength needs; for college football, however, 8 to 10 sets are more likely to produce significant strength gains.

Often, a major concern for the coach is time. Although more time spent strength training may produce significant strength gains, athletes may be unable to devote the time necessary for an intensive strength program. Many college athletes spend between 1½ to 3 hours training in weight rooms almost every day of the week. Your responsibility as a coach is to design programs that maximize the training effect and that can be realistically accomplished by your individual athletes.

To start an athlete on a strength program, it is better to begin with light weights, a few sets, and a high number of reps. At this stage it is essential that athletes learn the correct lifting techniques and are not overstressed. In its simplest form, a program might consist of 3 sets of 6 to 10 reps for each of your selected exercises. A sample program (ignoring sport specificity) is shown in Table 4.4.

Table 4.4
Sample Weight Training Program

Exercise	Reps[a]	Sets
Bench press	6-10	3
Half squat	6-10	3
Incline press	6-10	3
Toe raise	6-10	3
Sit-ups	10-20	3
Parallel bar dips	6-10	3
Wrist roller	6-10	3

[a]Once the athlete can perform the exercise 10 times, the weight may be increased by 5 to 10 lb (see guidelines in text for increasing weight).

The athlete would perform the series of exercises beginning with the bench press, completing 1 set, then continuing to the half squat. After completing all the exercises *once*, the athlete repeats the series two more times. This type of exercise circuit in which the reps and sets remain consistent will develop strength and will be easy for you to administer.

Varying the Training Program for Increased Strength Gains

As your athletes become more proficient, greater strength gains may be possible by introducing one of the many variations of this standard program. For example, you might start an athlete with a 1 RM bench press of 80 lb on a 3-set program in which the repetitions progressively decrease as the weight increases. The starting weight for bench press indicated in the previous chart serves as a warm-up weight. A beginning 3-set program would look like this:

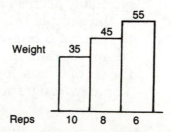

Depending on your athletes' abilities, you may need to use a barbell without a weight or even something a little lighter for the first set(s). Once it becomes evident that this is too easy, training intensity should be increased by adding sets and more weight. To develop strength, the general progression should be to reduce the number of reps and to increase the weight. Three sets is probably sufficient for most young athletes. For older, postpubescent athletes, you may want to consider increasing the number of sets, especially of the major exercises. Gradually, the athlete could be introduced into the following 8-set program for bench press:

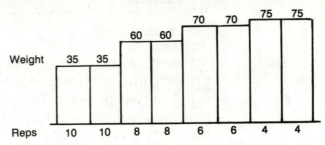

As your athletes attempt the programs you design, they will experience successes and failures. Be prepared to modify the program to ensure that each athlete is able to maintain a reasonable rate of progression. Let's suppose, for example, the athlete successfully completes the following planned 8-set series of reps:

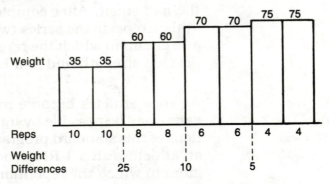

You will notice that the weight increases between each pair of sets (e.g., 10 & 8 sets, 8 & 6 sets, and 6 & 4 sets) were different. To adjust for these differences, a rule of thumb to remember is that the rate of increase should always be progressive, gradually decreasing as the load gets heavier. In other words, in the sample bench program, the coach might add 5 lb to the sets of 6 reps and 5 lb to the set of 4 reps. It would *not* be appropriate to add 15 lb to the set of 4 reps and 5 lb to the set of 6 reps, for this would upset the desired progression. The new program would look as follows:

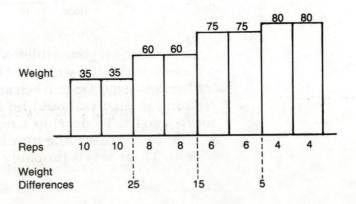

These principles of progression apply to all the exercises you might include in your strength program. With more experience and by observing the achievements of other coaches in your sport, you will be better able to organize effective strength programs for your athletes.

Circuit Training

Circuit training is an effective method for developing all the physical qualities inherent in muscular fitness. A circuit typically consists of 8 to 10 exercise areas where athletes perform either a specified number of repetitions or exercise for a certain period of time before moving immediately to the next exercise area. A circuit is completed when your athletes have performed each of the required exercises. Circuits can include weight training, variable resistance exercises, calisthenics, running, swimming, stretching, and most other forms of exercise.

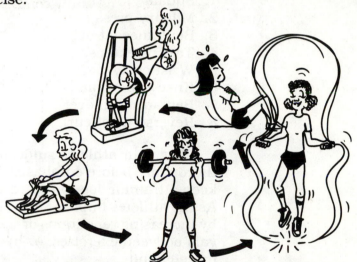

Circuit Design

By varying exercise selection, duration, and intensity, coaches can design circuits to meet the specific physical needs of their athletes. For an emphasis on strength, the program might consist entirely of weight training or variable resistance exercises; for an emphasis on endurance, running and calisthenics could also be included. Listed below are some general recommendations to be followed when designing a circuit.

- Alternate muscle groups to avoid local muscle fatigue; try to rotate from legs to trunk to arms to legs, and so on.
- Select exercises that simulate sport-specific movements and work the major muscle groups involved.
- For strength, follow strength training principles (6 to 10 RM).
- For power/endurance do 12 to 25 reps as fast as possible, then move to next station (or do 20 seconds, then move).

- Use weight machines to reduce risk of injury.
- Change less important exercises after several weeks to keep interest in the circuit.
- Start with one revolution of the circuit and build up to two or even three (for stronger, more experienced athletes).

Notice that these recommendations direct you to apply the principles already discussed for developing strength and endurance. Always try to select exercises based on the skills required in your sport and on the needs of your individual athletes. Shown below are two sample muscular fitness circuit training programs: the first for baseball, the second for basketball. (Exercises were selected from Table 4.3.)

Baseball Circuit	*Basketball Circuit*
1. Squats	1. Squats
2. Military press	2. Bench press
3. Bent-knee sit-ups	3. Heel raise
4. Triceps extension	4. Lateral arm raise
5. Wrist curl	5. Bent-knee sit-ups
6. Knee extension	6. Arm curl
7. Bent-arm pullover	7. Leg curl
8. Reverse wrist curl	8. Pulldown

Allow your athletes sufficient time to learn the exercises thoroughly before emphasizing speed. Each athlete should keep a training log to record weight, repetitions, and time. As the athletes improve, training intensity can be increased by increasing repetitions or weight, by decreasing rest intervals between exercises, or by having the athletes complete more circuits.

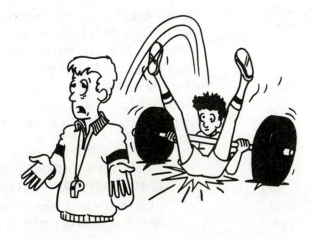

Safety

The use of free weights should be introduced with careful supervision and adequate spotting. Always encourage your athletes to train with at least one partner who can assist with carrying and changing weights and who will be ready to offer assistance if a load gets too heavy during exercise. For exercises involving heavy weights, *two* spotters are essential.

When setting up strength training programs for your athletes, teach them the proper lifting techniques and training procedures. Learning how to balance and handle heavy weights requires practice. Your athletes must understand the dangers of using incorrect or inappropriate techniques. Emphasize the dangers of holding competitions to see who can lift the greatest weight, and remind them that they are lifting weights to get stronger, not getting stronger to lift weights. Explain the differences between weight training and weight lifting. If your athletes are interested in competitive lifting, direct them to a class or club where they can receive expert instruction.

Before each training session, have your athletes go through a thorough warm-up. Be sure they are dressed properly; insist they wear rubber-soled shoes to protect the feet and to insure stability. Advise them to wear a weight belt when performing heavy weight training exercises. Belts help to prevent back and abdominal injuries.

Before your athletes begin, they should always check that the collars holding the weights on the bar are securely tightened. If they will be using other training devices, these also must be checked for hazards. When your athletes are exercising, encourage them to exhale during the lift and inhale as they lower the weight. Athletes should be able to handle the weight through a full range of motion. Do not let them try to lift weights that are too heavy, for this risks serious injury. Key safety recommendations are shown in the following safety checklist.

Weight Training Safety Checklist

- Assign two spotters when athletes are lifting heavy weights.
- Teach proper lifting and training techniques.
- Teach your athletes the dangers of incorrect techniques.
- Have your athletes warm up before lifting weights.
- Ensure that athletes are dressed properly and that they include a weight belt if performing heavy exercises.
- Teach athletes to check that collars are secure *before* lifting weights, along with checking safety features of other training devices.

Record Keeping

Each athlete should maintain a regular training log to record progress. Key features to record are the exercises and sets, weight or resistance and reps, and the date. A sample format for a beginning program is shown in Figure 4.1. Notice that the coach sets the weight and repetitions for each exercise. In the box below, a space is provided for the athlete to record the number of repetitions actually achieved. The coach and athlete are then able to compare training goals and achievements and to make any necessary adjustments to the program to ensure ongoing progression.

KEN BARNES
Athlete

FOOTBALL
Team

EDDY
Coach

Exercise	Dates						
	6/10	6/13	6/16	6/19	6/22	6/25	6/28
SQUATS	100/10	110/10	120/10	120/10			
	10	10	8	10			
BENCH PRESS	80/10	90/10	100/10	100/10			
	10	10	8	9			
KNEE EXTENSION	25/10	25/10	30/10	30/10			
	9	10	7	8			
HEEL RAISE	80/10	85/10	90/10	95/10			
	10	10	10	9			
LATERAL ARM RAISE	15/10	15/10	20/10	20/10			
	9	10	6	7			
BENT-KNEE SIT-UPS	30	35	40	45			
	30	35	40	42			
DIPS	10	10	10	12			
	8	9	10	10			

Figure 4.1. Weight training log.

For advanced training programs involving several different sets of the same exercise, many coaches prefer to record scores of only the major and assistant exercises. Shown in Figure 4.2 is a sample log for recording the scores of three exercises: bench press, squats, and incline press. Records are not kept for the supplementary and the specialty exercises in the training program. Athletes simply follow previously learned guidelines and consult regularly with the coach to ensure the correct progression.

Athlete: Mark Simon

Team: Wrestling

Date: _____

Coach: O'Brien

Bench	Squat	Incline	Bench	Squat	Incline
135×10	135×8	95×10	155×6		115×6
10	8	10	6		8
135×10	135×8	95×10	155×6		115×6
10	8	10	4		5
145×8	185×8	105×8	165×4		115×6
7	8	6	4		6
145×8	185×8	105×8	165×4		125×4
5	8	6	3		3
155×6	135×8	125×6			125×4
5	8	4			1
155×6	135×8	125×6			
4	8	2			
165×4	185×8	135×4			
3	8	2			
165×4	185×8	135×4			
2	8	2			
135×10	185×8	95×10			
10	8	10			
135×10		95×10			
10		10			
145×8		105×8			
8		8			
145×8		105×8			
8		8			

Figure 4.2. Advanced weight training log after two completed training sessions.

Rate of Improvement

Strength does not increase rapidly: 1% to 3% per week is an average rate of improvement although faster improvements (4% to 5%) may occur with hard training. Previously untrained muscles improve at a faster pace. During the strength program, your athletes should be prepared to meet and to overcome training plateaus. A lack of improvement is most visible if the 1 RM is the only estimate of strength. Although further improvements may not be apparent at this level, significant gains may be taking place at submaximal strength levels. Use the training log to point out to your athletes the improvements that are occurring at different strength levels.

Strength may increase 50% in 4 to 6 months; subsequent gains will come more slowly and require more time and effort. Strength improvements can continue beyond the age of 40, but the most dramatic improvements occur between puberty and 19. Strength will not improve so rapidly when it is combined with serious muscular endurance training. Do them separately for best results and build a solid strength foundation; then if endurance is a key quality in your sport, begin to emphasize endurance training principles.

Maintaining Strength

Studies show that athletes often lose strength during the competitive season. A maintenance program will ensure that strength is not neglected and will help your athletes keep their muscular fitness at a high level throughout the season. For most sports, during the playing season athletes can maintain strength with 1 to 2 training sessions per week.

In active individuals strength does not decline rapidly, but inactivity caused by illness or injury leads to more rapid strength loss. If any of your athletes must miss practice for more than a week, be sure they regain strength and endurance before returning to strenuous competition.

MUSCULAR ENDURANCE

In the past, sport physiologists believed that training with fewer than 10 reps produced strength and that more than 10 reps developed endurance. Recent studies have helped us expand that concept of endurance training, and we are now able to better match the exercise to its intended use.

Endurance Training Principles

Endurance training improves endurance in both slow- and fast-twitch muscle fibers. The various aspects of endurance, including short-term endurance, intermediate endurance, and long-term endurance, were discussed in chapter 3. Short-term endurance training will improve strength as well as the ability to sustain effort against a moderately high resistance (e.g., an opponent's body in wrestling). Intermediate endurance training provides endurance for lesser loads, such as an athlete's own body weight in basketball. Finally, long-term endurance training improves the production of energy and the oxygen utilization that is needed for prolonged exertion with a low resistance (e.g., in distance running). Shown in Table 4.5 are training guidelines for developing these different types of endurance.

Ensure that athletes follow the recommendations for each muscle group being trained. Increase the sets and times per week for advanced training. For sports that require long-term endurance, encourage long duration training sessions.

Table 4.5
Endurance Training Guidelines

	Repetitions	Sets	Times/Week
Short-term endurance	15-25	3	3
Intermediate endurance	30-50	2	3
Long-term endurance[a]	100+	1	3

[a]Also includes numerous low-resistance contractions in movements that are specific to the sport.

The physiological effects of varying the number of repetitions and the sports likely to profit from each method are shown in Table 4.6. As resistance decreases (or reps increase), you move from an emphasis on strength training to endurance training. Although the effects of training do overlap, an emphasis on either strength training or long-term endurance training will have distinctly different outcomes. Coaches must first identify individual needs, then plan a training program to meet those specific needs.

Endurance Training Methods

Short-term and intermediate endurance can be gained using weights, weight machines, calisthenics, or special training devices designed to suit the sport. Perhaps you can design your own sport-specific training centers or training devices. (The low-cost backyard training center I built for cross-country skiing training provides an endurance training circuit for my son and me that exercises many of the muscle groups used in the sport.) If you do decide to develop an endurance training machine, remember to apply the principle of specificity and to select exercises that closely simulate the movements of the sport. With a little thought you may be able to develop some unique training methods that will benefit your athletes.

Table 4.6
Physiological Effects of Varying Exercise Repetitions

	Strength	Short-Term Endurance	Intermediate Endurance	Long-Term Endurance
Types of training	High resistance 6-8 RM[a]	Medium/high resistance 12-25 RM	Medium resistance 30-50 RM	Low resistance 100+ RM[b]
Effects of training	Size of muscle and connective tissue increases Contractile protein increases Short-term energy increases Neuromuscular skill increases Inhibitions decrease	Strength and short-term energy increases Work output increases Neuromuscular skill increases	Some endurance and short-term energy increases Work output increases Neuromuscular efficiency increases	Oxygen-using enzymes in endurance energy pathways increase Capillaries increase Long-term energy increases Neuromuscular efficiency increases
Sports	Short/intense Heavy loads Football Shot, discus Weight lifting	Medium/high load and duration Wrestling Hockey Boxing	Moderate intensity load and duration Basketball Soccer Field hockey	Long duration, low intensity Distance running Swimming Cycling Cross-country skiing

[a]RM = Repetitions Maximum—the most you can do.
[b]Include numerous low-resistance contractions.

**Organizing
an Endurance
Training Program**

Much of the advice given in the strength training section applies to endurance. Similar exercises can be used, and identical safety procedures should be enforced. The training log shown in Figure 4.1 is ideal for endurance training.

The main organizational difference is the starting point of the program. To be able to perform the number of repetitions advised for developing endurance, a slightly lighter starting weight must be used. Experimentation will enable you to discover the correct figure, though it will probably be 50 to 75% of the 1 RM figure.

**Rate
of Improvement**

Although it may take months to improve strength by 50%, it is possible to go from 20 to 30 push-ups in a few days. Part of this improvement can be attributed to increased skill, but research has shown that endurance can improve at an astonishing rate. In one study, the subjects lifted a 25-lb weight at a set cadence. Before training, 30 reps was an average score. After 2 months, some subjects were doing over 1,000 reps! Muscular endurance remains trainable into middle age and beyond. Many previously sedentary middle-aged individuals have become national caliber age group athletes in endurance sports.

Another study at the University of Montana Human Performance Laboratory showed a 75% increase in work output after 8 weeks of short-term endurance training (15 to 25 RM). With long-term endurance training, the improvements can be phenomenal. Although it is hard to generalize about rates of progress, studies have shown that young athletes who do push-ups regularly for 10 weeks might improve from 20 to 60 reps, a threefold, or 300% improvement. This represents an improvement of 30% per week. As the athlete approaches some upper limit dictated by heredity (fiber type, etc.), the rate of improvement will decrease but will often have a more significant effect on performance than gains in strength.

**Maintaining
Endurance**

One of your key responsibilities as a coach is to help your athletes maintain the physical capabilities they need for successful skill performance. In general, short-term endurance is easier to maintain. The muscle enzymes produced in long-term endurance training are quickly lost during periods of inactivity. One study has shown that long-term endurance is lost three times faster than it is gained. Healthy subjects improved 3% per week in training but lost 9% each week they spent in bed. Once your athletes have improved their muscular endurance, they must work out regularly—two to three times a week—to keep it. Although athletes will only lose 4% of their endurance per week if they stay regularly active, be sure to continue endurance training during the competitive season to avoid any loss.

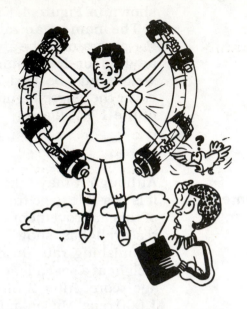

POWER

Power depends on the effective combination of strength and speed and on short-term energy sources and pathways. An improvement of either strength or speed will increase power.

Power Training Principles

When training specifically for power, your athletes must attempt to move a load as fast as possible. Power training enhances strength, speed, and energy supplies. Guidelines for developing power are shown in Table 4.7.

Table 4.7
Power Training Guidelines

	Repetitions[a]	Sets	Times/Week
Power	15-25 RM[b]	3	3

[a]Speed: As fast as possible.
[b]Resistance should be 30 to 60% of maximum strength.

When you select exercises for a power training program, remember to pattern them after the movements in the sport. The speed of exercise should closely match the speed of the sport-specific movements. Use less resistance (30% of max) for low-resistance activities, such as throwing a baseball, and more resistance for heavy resistance sports, such as blocking in football. The blocking sled used in football is an ideal way to train for power. The resistance is relatively high, and the team can do the movement as fast as possible with minimal risk of injury.

Power Training Methods

Because power is so closely related to strength, it can be developed using similar training methods. Free weights, weight machines, variable resistance devices, and other specially designed training equipment all lend themselves to power training. Circuit training that emphasizes speed is especially effective. Exercise selection and speed of muscle contraction are the two variables that the coach must control to stimulate improvements in power.

Preload

Another way to develop power is by utilizing the preload and elastic recoil present in many sport skills. In running, for example, the strong thigh muscles of the leg are slightly stretched or preloaded before they contract to drive the runner forward. The stretch stores up elastic energy that is quickly released during the contraction. Similarly, as a tennis player begins the backswing for a forehand, the triceps muscle on the back of the upper arm contracts, and the biceps muscle on the front of the arm stretches. When the player begins to swing forward, the biceps contracts powerfully in response to its rapid stretching. This extra power does not take much extra energy, so it provides more power without any added cost, a true example of efficiency. The same principle can be applied in such movements as throwing the javelin or discus and in jumping, as well as in other sports where a brief stretch can be quickly followed by a contraction. A group of training methods that apply this principle to develop power are sometimes known as *plyometrics*.

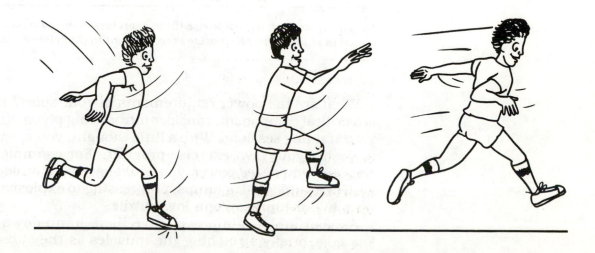

Plyometrics

European athletes have long used plyometrics—explosive calisthenic-like exercises—to develop power. A key feature of plyometric training is the conditioning of the neuromuscular system to permit faster and more powerful changes of direction, such as moving from down to up in jumping or switching leg positions as in running. Reducing the time needed for this change in direction increases speed and power.

Ski jumpers, cross-country and downhill skiers, basketball and volleyball players, sprinters, high jumpers, and other athletes who require power can profit from plyometric training. In addition to being effective, plyometric exercises are relatively easy to teach and learn. Plyometric exercises utilize the following movements: bounds, hops, jumps, leaps, skips, ricochets, swings, and twists.

A sample program of plyometric exercises for different muscle groups is shown in Table 4.8. A typical plyometric program will have 8 to 10 reps, 3 to 5 sets, and a rest interval of 1 to 2 min between each set. A description of these exercises is included in Appendix C.

Table 4.8
Sample Plyometric Training Program[a]

Muscle Groups	Exercises
Legs and hips	Double leg bound
	Alternate leg bound
	Double leg speed hop
	Squat jump
	Split jump
	Skipping
Trunk	Floor kip
	Medicine ball twist/toss
Upper body	Medicine ball chest pass
	Heavy bag thrust

[a]A full explanation of how to use these exercises to develop power is contained in *Plyometrics: Explosive Power Training* (Radcliffe & Farentinos, 1985).

What are the power requirements in your sport? If power is a critical component, consider introducing plyometrics into your training sessions. With a little thought, you may be able to design your own exercise program. For example, if you want to improve leg power, you could have your athletes start with one- and two-leg jumps, progressing to explosive jumps up a hill or jumps over a low hurdle.

As your athletes improve, have them jump down from a low box, briefly stretching the muscles as they absorb the shock, and then explode upward, employing muscle preload and elastic recoil for added power. Because body weight is about 33% of max leg strength, plyometrics fit the power training prescription. Just be sure to start athletes gradually and do all jumping on grass or mats to avoid unnecessary soreness. Because plyometrics place considerable stress on the joint structures, observe your athletes' reaction closely. Athletes who begin to complain of soreness or pain around the joints should avoid plyometrics.

Organizing a Power Training Program

Weight training and variable resistance are both suitable for developing power. The advice on exercise selection and safety and on keeping a training log given in the previous two sections is applicable for power. The principal difference will be in the speed with which the exercises are performed.

With variable resistance devices this is easy because resistance is controlled by the machine and depends on the speed of the muscle contraction. Athletes simply aim to perform as fast as possible. Developing power with weights requires some experimentation to identify a load the athlete can move quickly for the desired number of repetitions.

Rate of Improvement

Improvements in power are rapid in the first month because most athletes have never trained specifically for power. When the rate of improvement begins to level off or reach a plateau, further improvement is possible by (a) concentrating on specific strength training, (b) concentrating on specific speed training, or (c) increasing resistance or repetitions in the power training program. Deciding among these choices depends on the nature of the sport you coach: Increase resistance for high-resistance sports like football, and increase speed or repetitions for low-resistance events like cross-country skiing.

Maintaining Power

Energy stores and enzymes associated with power are lost rather quickly, so you must continue a maintenance program—at least once a week—throughout the season. Because power and strength maintenance does not require many sets, both can be accomplished in a reasonably short session. Be sure to maintain strength and power in the muscle groups essential for skill performance and injury prevention in your sport.

If power is important in your sport, schedule maintenance on light training days, as far away from the next competition as possible. This maintains the rhythm of training while providing a nice diversion from the typical practice session. Power declines rapidly with age and with an inevitable decrease in rapid activity. Because older individuals seldom do rapid, forceful contractions, they lose power before they lose strength and endurance.

SPEED

The final and perhaps most elusive muscular fitness component we will consider is speed. Improving the speed of your athletes, although often highly desirable, depends not only on the athletes' willingness to train but also on genetically determined muscular characteristics.

Speed Training Principles

Fast-twitch fibers provide more speed than slow-twitch muscle. Athletes with a high proportion of fast-twitch fibers will enjoy a natural speed advantage over athletes with a predominant quantity of slow-twitch fibers. However, studies have shown that the neuromuscular apparatus can be taught to do complex skills at a faster rate. The key to improving speed is to practice the movements at faster than normal speeds; this helps the nervous system to overcome inhibitions and to learn to perform at a faster pace.

In a few sports excessive speed can be counterproductive, especially if accompanied by poor technique. Move the hands too fast in swimming or the oar too fast in rowing and you lose your "grip" on the water. Improvement of technique should precede any training emphasis on increasing speed. Focus on speed *only* when you are confident in your athlete's skills. However, it is true that in most sports, differences in speed have a significant impact on performance, and athletes can profit from specific speed training.

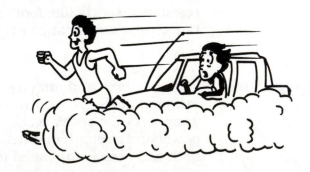

Speed Training Methods

Speed training should be founded on a comprehensive program of strength, endurance, and power development. Preseason and early season training must focus on the improvement of these basic components of muscular fitness. As the competitive season approaches, specific speed work can be integrated into daily practices.

Climatic conditions should be considered when speed training. Rushing into speed work during cold weather can have disastrous results. If you must do sprints in cold weather, insist on a good warm-up and make sure the athletes wear warm clothing.

Because the principle of speed training is to perform sport-specific movements at a faster than usual pace, the task of the coach is to (a) identify the crucial movement patterns in his or her sport, and (b) select training methods that will help the athlete perform these movements faster. In a sport like baseball where pitching speed is vital, coaches should emphasize speed as soon as the muscles are conditioned and ready for high-intensity work. A weighted ball in the off-season might further enhance speed.

In high velocity events such as sprints and the long jump, coaches must emphasize power and speed as soon as muscles are ready. One method is to have your athletes try running down a slight grade as fast as they dare. Alternatively, coach your athletes to perform a movement as fast as possible. This idea might work well for athletes involved in combat sports. At first their movements will be sloppy, but in time the neuromuscular apparatus will adjust, and they will enjoy an advantage over slower opponents.

Rate of Improvement

In addition to improvements in the neuromuscular apparatus, speed training increases short-term energy, the energy used during the first seconds of all-out effort. A well-learned skill isn't quickly lost, but the energy stores only remain elevated during a period of intense training. It takes about 6 weeks of intense training to elevate this energy, so most coaches recommend using the weeks preceding the peak season to put the final touches on speed and on short-term energy stores.

SUMMARY

1. Specificity of training is the most important principle to apply to all training methods. Coaches must consider the specific needs of their sport and their athletes when selecting training methods and when organizing a muscular fitness program.

2. By varying exercise intensity, duration, and frequency, coaches are able to control the training emphasis.

3. Flexibility exercises should be included in the warm-up that begins every training program. Because flexibility declines with age, athletes should be encouraged to maintain flexibility throughout the year.

4. Isometrics (static contractions), isotonics (weight training), isokinetics (variable resistance), calisthenics,

and plyometrics are the major training methods for developing strength, endurance, power, and speed.

5. Circuit training is an effective method of organizing selected exercises into a training program.

6. Optimal strength development occurs with 6 to 10 reps repeated at least 3 times. Greater repetitions will stimulate improvements in muscular endurance.

7. Power is effectively developed by moving a resistance as fast as possible.

8. Speed improvement is possible by performing sport-specific movements at a faster than usual pace.

Training guidelines for each of the elements that contribute to muscular fitness are shown in Table 4.9.

These training methods must be integrated into a total fitness program for your athletes and will be discussed in chapter 8. But first, let's consider the other major fitness component—*energy fitness*.

Table 4.9
Muscular Fitness Training Guidelines

	Maximum Repetitions (RM)	Sets	Times/Week
Strength			
Weights	6-8 RM	3[a]	3
Isokinetic exercises			
Slow	8	3	3
Fast	15	3	3
Calisthenics	6-8 RM	3	3
Endurance			
Short-term	15-25 RM	3	3
Intermediate	30-50 RM	2	3
Long-term	100+[b]	1	3
Power			
Less resistance— 30% max FAP	15-25 RM[c]	3	3
More resistance— 60% max FAP	10-15 RM[c]	3	3

[a]Increase, after 8 to 12 weeks, to 4 and eventually 5 sets.

[b]As in running, cycling, swimming, and cross-country skiing.

[c]Fast as possible.

PART 3
Training for Energy Fitness

Chapter 5
Energy Systems

In this chapter the energy systems that power muscular movements will be examined. Depending on the intensity of the exercise, the body can draw on several sources of energy. Exercise intensity also determines the recruitment of slow-twitch or fast-twitch muscle fibers. The different muscle fiber types rely on different energy systems and each is uniquely suited for certain types of movement.

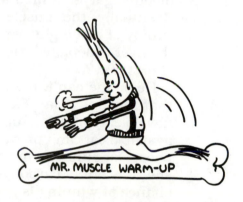

MR. MUSCLE WARM-UP

TYPES OF ENERGY SYSTEMS

Imagine that you are able to observe a muscle fiber just before the start of a race. The fiber has been warmed up, stretched, and now awaits the sound of the gun. The gun fires and as the athlete begins running, you observe the vigorous contracting and relaxing of the fiber. The energy for contraction comes from two compounds stored and ready for use in the muscle. These compounds, *Adenosine Triphosphate* (ATP) and *Creatine Phosphate* (CP), are in limited supply, so if something doesn't happen soon, the muscle will run out of them. After about 10 seconds of exercise, just as ATP and CP are running low, an answer to the energy need appears when the muscle starts to use *glycogen* (stored carbohydrate) to produce more ATP. About this time, a by-product produced during the breaking down glycogen, *lactic acid*, begins to appear in the muscle cells. Unfortunately, acidic by-products can inhibit energy production. If a solution doesn't appear quickly, the muscle will not be able to continue.

After a couple of minutes, just when things are looking grim, the muscle gets its second wind from a supply of oxygen that allows the efficient use of both carbohydrate and fat to produce ATP. Why wasn't the oxygen there from the start? The onset of exercise triggers an increase in respiration and circulation that is designed to bring oxygen and fuel to the muscle and to take carbon dioxide and lactic acid away. Although the heart and lungs increase their output gradually, it takes about 2 minutes to transport the needed oxygen to the working muscles. Then and only then can the muscle fibers produce energy efficiently.

As the race continues, you will observe that the ratio of carbohydrate to fat utilization varies with the intensity of effort. As the runner speeds up or runs up hills, he or she uses a greater proportion of carbohydrate. On the downhills, when less energy is needed, the proportion of carbohydrate declines. When he or she sprints to pass another runner, the muscle shifts completely to carbohydrate for energy. As the race continues, the muscle glycogen supply dwindles, but suddenly, a new supply of carbohydrate enters the muscle. This new supply, *blood glucose* (blood sugar), can fill in for a while, but blood sugar is limited and needed by the nervous system. Eventually, the muscle carbohydrate is exhausted and the supply of blood glucose is reduced as the limited supply in the liver is depleted. How can the runner keep up his or her efforts now?

He or she can't, not in this race. The only energy source that remains is fat. Fat is a great source of energy, and we have plenty of it, but, unfortunately, when carbohydrate isn't available, fat can't produce energy fast enough to sustain race pace. Our runner can walk or jog slowly on fat, but if he or she runs out of carbohydrate before the end of the race, the chance of winning is gone; he or she may even be lucky to finish.

What about protein as an energy source? Protein is not used very much as a fuel for exercise unless you are on a low-calorie diet. The body prefers to use the other energy sources and to conserve protein to make tissue, enzymes, and other important compounds. Athletes should never approach competition on a low-calorie or starvation diet, because although this may help them lose weight, they will also experience a loss of strength and endurance due to lack of energy supplies.

SOURCES OF ENERGY

ATP and CP, the immediate sources of energy for muscular contractions, are stored in resting muscles ready for instant use. Unfortunately, they are also in short supply, providing for only seconds of all-out effort. For this reason ATP and CP are called short-term energy supplies. Athletes rely on short-term energy supplies at the start of effort and whenever the pace is increased. Otherwise, exercise is fueled by the metabolism (breakdown) of carbohydrate and fat to produce

ATP energy. The various sources of energy used during exercise are illustrated in Figure 5.1.

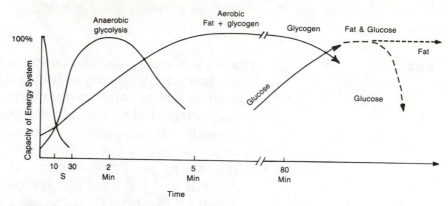

Figure 5.1. Energy production during exercise. As muscle glycogen is used up, blood glucose temporarily fills the demand for carbohydrate.

Carbohydrate

Carbohydrate is eaten in the form of starches (i.e., potatoes, rice, corn, beans, whole grain products) or simple sugars (i.e., table sugar, honey). The starches are broken into the simple sugars for digestion, then the sugar is stored in the liver (about 80 g) and is used to restock the muscle glycogen supply (about 15 g/kg of muscle in the untrained athlete). If your athletes eat more sugar than is needed to restock the liver and muscles, the excess sugar is converted to fat and stored in adipose tissue storage depots. Some of this blood sugar is also used immediately by the body for energy. The brain and nervous system rely on blood glucose as an energy source, and low blood glucose levels—a condition called hypoglycemia—can affect the function of the brain and the nervous system.

The total supply of carbohydrate in muscles, liver, and blood (shown in Table 5.1) is enough to fuel a 10-mile run.

Table 5.1
Total Carbohydrate Energy for Adolescents

Source	Amount in Grams	Calories[a]
Liver[b]	80 g	320
Blood	4 g	16
Muscle (20 kg)	15 g/kg = 300 g	1,200
	TOTAL =	1,536 cal

[a]It takes 5 cal/min to walk, 10 cal/min to jog, and over 20 cal/min to run fast. About 110 cal are used running a mile.

[b]Much of the carbohydrate stored in the liver and carried in the blood is needed by the brain and nervous system.

For longer endurance activities, it pays to increase muscle glycogen storage. This can be accomplished by eating a high-carbohydrate diet several days before the event—a process known as carbohydrate loading.

Fat

The fat you eat is absorbed and carried to the tissues of the body. Some may be used as fuel and some may go to the liver for conversion to other compounds. But much of the excess fat is transported to the adipose tissue for storage where it stays until it is used to fuel muscular contractions. Fat is our primary source of stored fuel; it carries more than twice as much energy per gram as carbohydrate, yielding 9 cal/g as compared to 4 cal/g for carbohydrate.

When we exercise, fat is released from storage and used as a fuel to provide more ATP. Because most of us have at least 50 times more energy in fat than carbohydrate, we should learn to conserve carbohydrates and use fat whenever possible. Not only does this increase endurance, but it is good for our health; it means that the fat will be burned instead of ending up in the coronary arteries and causing a heart attack.

A problem with fat is that we do not use it much during extremely vigorous exercise. Because it takes more oxygen to burn fat, the body switches over to carbohydrate as exercise becomes more intense (see Figure 5.2). The right kind of physical training, however, will increase the muscle fiber's ability to use oxygen to burn fat. Several months of training teaches the body to use more fat and less carbohydrate to fuel a particular rate of exercise, for example, running at a pace of 6 min/mi. With training, endurance improves significantly, as muscles shift over to the inexhaustible supply of fat energy.

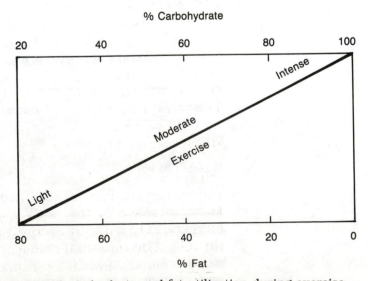

Figure 5.2. Carbohydrate and fat utilization during exercise.

After several months of training, athletes who could not run a mile at the start of training, discover they can run 20 or more.

ANAEROBIC AND AEROBIC ENERGY SYSTEMS

The anaerobic and aerobic systems are the major energy systems. The difference between the two is that the anaerobic systems do not use oxygen to break down carbohydrates, whereas the aerobic system uses oxygen to produce energy from carbohydrate and fat. At the start of exercise the body uses the anaerobic systems.

Anaerobic Systems

There are two anaerobic systems: stored ATP and CP, and anaerobic glycogen breakdown (*anaerobic glycolysis*). The energy at the start of exercise and whenever effort is increased comes from stored ATP and CP. During exercise, fuel is supplied by ATP produced from carbohydrate or fat metabolism. The anaerobic breakdown of stored muscle glycogen produces a small amount of ATP energy and the metabolic by-product lactic acid. Energy supplied by this system is important in events that require all-out effort for up to 4 minutes. This process was illustrated in Figure 5.1.

Aerobic System

Aerobic means with oxygen. The aerobic energy system uses oxygen in the breakdown of carbohydrate and fat to produce energy efficiently. The same carbohydrate molecule that yields 3 molecules of ATP and lactic acid without oxygen will produce 39 molecules of ATP with oxygen. Because of this difference, it is easy to understand why aerobic exercise feels easy, effortless, and economical, whereas anaerobic effort is so difficult and limited in time. Inside the muscle cell, carbohydrate in the form of glucose combines with oxygen to form carbon dioxide, water, and energy.

Aerobic, or oxygen-using, enzymes, which are located in the *mitochondria* (in the muscle cells), chip away at the carbohydrate molecule, releasing its stored energy. One effect of endurance training is that it increases the size and number of mitochondria, which increases the concentration and activity of the aerobic enzymes. This means that endurance-trained muscles become better able to use oxygen for energy production. As a result, carbohydrate metabolism is far more efficient, and the muscle is able to use more fat, thereby conserving the limited supply of muscle glycogen. The result is an increase in the body's ability to utilize or consume oxygen ($\dot{V}O_2$) without becoming fatigued and producing lactic acid. The maximal rate at which the body can consume oxygen for the production of energy is called the maximal aerobic power, or $\dot{V}O_2max$.

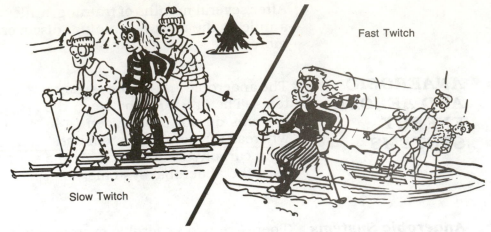

Fast Twitch

Slow Twitch

FIBER TYPES AND THEIR SPECIFIC ENERGY SYSTEMS

Each muscle fiber type is particularly well suited for certain types of exercise, and each has its own predominant energy system. Slow-twitch fibers (slow oxidative), which were described in chapter 3 on muscular fitness, are well supplied with aerobic enzymes. These fibers are used for slower, longer activities like jogging. Fast oxidative glycolytic (FOG) fibers have the capability for fast contractions, but they also have some endurance qualities. Fast glycolytic (FG) fibers are best suited for fast, short efforts. The fibers used by the body depend upon the intensity of physical activity as measured by the amount of oxygen (% $\dot{V}O_2$) being consumed during the activity. This process is illustrated in Figure 5.3.

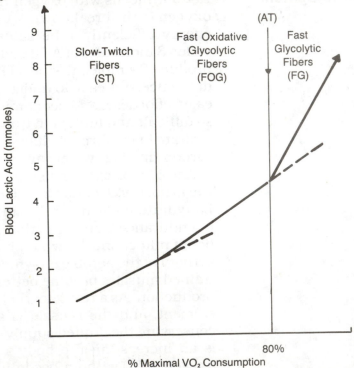

Figure 5.3. The anaerobic threshold (AT) (also called onset of blood lactic acid [OBLA], lactate threshold, or ventilatory threshold). Slow fibers are recruited for light work, fast-twitch fibers are added for more vigorous effort. (Adapted from Skinner & McLellan, 1980.)

At a slow jog, the body uses slow fibers. As the athlete speeds up, FOG fibers, then FG fibers are recruited into action. When designing a training program for your athletes, you must consider the effects of training on the fiber types and their energy systems, and on the physical demands of the sport. Athletes in short-duration events should concentrate on training their fast-twitch muscle fibers. For events of longer duration, athletes must develop the aerobic or endurance potential of both slow-twitch and FOG fibers. Remember, even in endurance events, well-trained slow-twitch fibers need help from fast-twitch fibers to go fast and kick at the end of the race.

Shown in Figure 5.3 is the rate of formation of lactic acid that occurs as speed is increased during a run. During a slow run, little lactic acid is produced by the slow fibers. As speed increases and as FOG fibers begin to be used, lactic acid forms faster. Even more speed produces a dramatic rise in lactic acid, a sign that the FG fibers are working. The transition to FG fibers, a stage in which lactic acid begins to accumulate rapidly, is the *anaerobic threshold* (sometimes referred to as the *lactate threshold*). The rapid rise in lactic acid limits the continuation of exercise as acidic by-products accumulate and inhibit energy production and contraction.

Training below this threshold will improve the aerobic energy systems. When exercise intensity rises above the anaerobic threshold, training enhances the capacity of anaerobic energy systems.

SUMMARY

1. Adenosine Triphosphate (ATP) and Creatine Phosphate (CP), which are stored in resting muscles, are the immediate sources of energy for muscular contractions.

2. As activity continues, additional ATP is provided by the anaerobic breakdown of stored muscle glycogen.

3. This process, however, also produces lactic acid, an acidic by-product that impedes the continuation of activity.

4. As soon as the respiratory and circulatory systems have adjusted to the muscles' need for oxygen, the aerobic breakdown of carbohydrate and fat provides ATP for ongoing activity, and the unwanted lactic acid may be removed by less active muscles.

5. Although fat is our primary source of stored fuel, carbohydrate is the principal source of energy during intense physical activity.

6. Slow-twitch and fast-twitch muscle fibers are ideally suited for specific types of activity, and each fiber type has its own predominant energy system.

7. Training should concentrate on improving the energy systems of the specific muscle fibers used when performing a sport.

8. As exercise intensity increases, there is a transition from the use of slow-twitch fibers to the use of slow-twitch and fast oxidative glycolytic fibers (FOG); finally, fast glycolytic fibers (FG) join in. The transitory phase from FOG fibers to FG fibers may be associated with the anaerobic, or lactate threshold.

In the next chapter you will learn how to determine the correct intensity of exercise to achieve desired changes in energy systems and muscle fibers that will improve the performances of your athletes.

Chapter 6
Energy Fitness Training

Coaches are like physicians: First, they diagnose an athlete's condition to determine what is needed; then they prescribe a training program to help the athlete meet the demands of the sport. Training stimulates a specific response in the body; and as with other treatments or drugs, the dosage must be prescribed with care. Just the right dose leads to the desired adaptations: Too little and the changes won't occur; too much and athletes risk the perils of overtraining—injury or illness. Good training programs are scientifically designed to bring about improvements in energy supplies, energy pathways, and muscle fibers. As energy training progresses, improvements also take place in important supply and support systems, including respiration, the blood, heart, and circulation. Tendons, ligaments, and bones become tougher as well. The hormones and the nervous system become more efficient, which leads to improved performance and various psychological benefits. Energy training can even lower blood fats and reduce the risk of heart disease. However, although a moderate amount of training is good for health, the hard-working athlete frequently walks a fine line between healthy training and overtraining. A wisely designed energy training program is a safeguard against the problems caused by overtraining.

ENERGY TRAINING PRINCIPLES

In the section on strength training, the principles of overload, adaptation, and progression were emphasized. These principles are equally applicable when training the energy systems and can be controlled by attending to the same three training variables: intensity, duration, and frequency. Intensity is the most important factor for controlling energy training. When training for strength, you can control intensity by varying the training load and exercise duration. For energy fitness, you control exercise intensity by having your athletes monitor their heart rates. As your athletes' heart rates increase during exercise, this indicates a gradual transition from aerobic (oxidative) to anaerobic (nonoxidative) energy pathways. The heart rate also indicates the body's transition from fat to carbohydrate energy and the recruitment of more fast-twitch muscle fibers. Let's examine more closely how your athletes can use their heart rate to control exercise intensity.

HEART RATE

The rate of the heart beat is controlled by a center in the brain. This center speeds up or slows down the heart according to information received from muscles and sensors located throughout the body. During exercise, when the muscles need more oxygen, the heart rate accelerates. You can count the heart rate by placing your fingers below your left breast. A more convenient technique is to count the pulse at the wrist where the radial artery is located. Simply lay your right hand in your left palm, face up, then slide the fingers of your left hand down the right thumb to the wrist and find the pulse in the groove above (or up the arm from) the thumb. Once you can do this proficiently, show your athletes how they can do it, too.

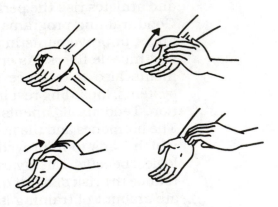

Resting Heart Rate

The resting heart rate is a good guide to the state of training. With better conditioning, the resting heart rate usually declines from the average of 70 beats per minute (bpm). Mine is under 50 when I'm in good shape, and I've seen some in the low 30s. Recording day-to-day heart rate variations will enable your athletes to monitor changes in their fitness and health.

Have your athletes take their resting heart rate every morning before rising. They will find it is higher when they are not feeling well or when they have a fever. Athletes who don't feel well and have a resting rate more than 5 beats above normal should consider an easy workout or a day off from training. They may be overtired or coming down with a cold, and a day of rest could hasten their recovery.

Maximal Heart Rate

Just as each of us has our own resting heart rate, we have a maximal heart rate as well. The maximal rate is what you'd expect—the highest your heart rate will go. Last time I checked mine it was 180 bpm. You can estimate your rate with this formula:

$$\text{Max HR} = 220 - \text{your age}$$

According to this formula, a 16-year-old athlete will have an estimated maximal heart rate of 204. As the formula also indicates, the maximum heart rate declines with age (see Figure 6.1). Because my maximal heart rate is 180 bpm, you might guess that I am 40 years old. You'd be wrong, however; I'm older than that. But this does raise an interesting point about the maximum heart rate—the rate of decline with age is slower in more active individuals. You should also know that highly trained young endurance athletes usually average lower maximal rates than their less active friends. If you coach highly trained young endurance athletes, use the following formula to calculate their maximum heart rate:

$$\text{Max HR} = 210 - \text{their age}$$

If you are interested in a precise measurement of your athletes' maximum HR, you can have them take an electrocardiogram-monitored exercise test on a treadmill or bicycle. If this is possible, be sure the athlete continues as long as possible; otherwise, you will not get a maximal value. Another way is to have athletes determine their max HR by running up a long, gradual hill for at least 6 to 8 minutes. Tell them to increase their pace gradually until they are going as fast as they can. They should keep pushing until they have to slow down, then stop and immediately check their rate (15 s rate × 4 or 6 s rate × 10 = bpm). Just be sure the athletes are in good condition before you attempt this test.

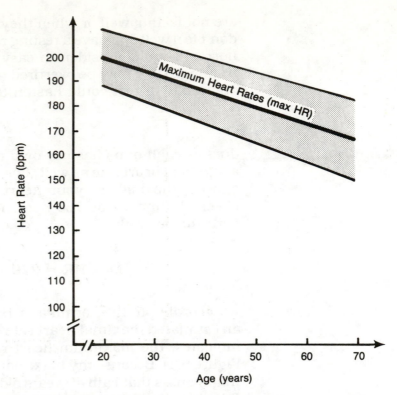

Figure 6.1. The average maximum heart rate. The maximum heart rate declines with age. The shaded area indicates the variability in this measurement. Some are 12 beats or more above or below the average for a given age.

**Training
Heart Rate**

The training heart rate is best found by placing your fingers *lightly* along the throat just to the side of the windpipe. The beat is particularly strong here during or just after exercise. The training heart rate is the best indicator of exercise intensity, for it is closely related to the amount of blood being pumped, the amount of oxygen being used, and the number of calories being burned. The relationship is so precise that it forms a straight line, allowing one to be predicted from the other. This relationship is shown in Figure 6.2.

As the training heart rate goes up, it indicates a gradual switch from fat to carbohydrate as a source of energy. As it goes even higher, it coincides with a gradual shift from aerobic to anaerobic energy production. Also, because the body uses slow-muscle fibers for slow activity and both slow and fast fibers for faster effort, the rising training heart rate coincides with recruitment of fast-twitch fibers. The training heart rate is an effective method of controlling exercise intensity and of ensuring that your athletes are training correctly.

**CONTROLLING
TRAINING
INTENSITY**

Because the training heart rate is your way of gauging the intensity of training, it helps answer concerns such as, "Are my athletes training fast enough?" "Are they going too fast?"

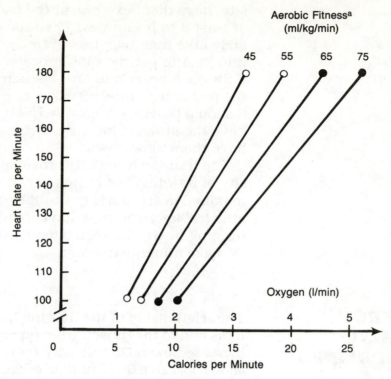

Figure 6.2. Predicting oxygen intake and calories burned during physical activity from the heart rate. Find the line that approximates your athletes' aerobic fitness. Read across from the exercise heart rate, then down to determine oxygen intake and calories burned. A runner with a 165 heart rate and a 65 (ml/kg/min) fitness score will be burning approximately 20 cal/min (1,200/hr).

[a]See chapter 7 for a test of aerobic fitness.

Note. 15-s pulse count taken immediately after exercise (15-s rate × 4 = rate/min). (Adapted from Sharkey, 1974, 1975.)

By using the training heart rate to guide each phase of training, you can be assured your athletes will be doing the right thing for their energy sources, energy pathways, and muscle fiber types.

For all sports, the early stages of energy training call for slow, easy endurance work. For athletes in average physical condition, a training intensity of 70 to 85% of the athlete's maximum HR is probably appropriate. As as example, consider Steven, a skier who has a maximum HR of 200 bpm. His coach Bob knows that he must build up to the season and must do so at the correct intensity to make steady progress. Bob uses the following equations to determine the range of Steven's exercising heart rate.

$$\text{Max HR} = 200 \times 70\% = 140 \text{ bpm}$$
$$\text{Max HR} = 200 \times 85\% = 170 \text{ bpm}$$

If Steven trains within this range (140 to 170 bpm), he will achieve his early season training goals.

To be sure that your athletes' heart rates are in the correct range and that your athletes are training at the right intensity, have them exercise at the pace you think is correct for at least 3 to 5 minutes. Then have them stop and immediately take their own heart rate for 15 seconds. Multiply this rate by 4 to get the rate in beats per minute. For example, if Steven's heart rate for 15 seconds was 38 after skiing for the prescribed time, his heart rate is 152 bpm—right where it should be (HR = 38 × 4 = 152 bpm). If the rate is too slow, have the athletes increase their pace a bit. If it is too high, have them slow down.

The training heart rate provides a way to gauge the intensity of training, but remember, it is only an estimate. If the maximal heart rate is quite different than the average for an athletes' age, you may have to adjust this guideline. If the training heart rate seems too hard or too easy, be prepared to make an adjustment.

ENERGY TRAINING GUIDELINES

The relationship of the training heart rate to the energy systems and to the muscle fiber types, and the training effect of increased exercise intensity on these systems and fibers is shown in Table 6.1. Duration of training will be discussed later in this chapter.

Table 6.1
Heart Rate Training Guides[a]

% Max HR	HR[b]	Training Effect
60-80%	120-160	Aerobic energy sources Aerobic energy pathways Slow-twitch muscle fibers
80-90%	160-180	Aerobic energy pathways Slow-twitch and FOG fibers Anaerobic (or lactate) threshold
90-95%	180-190	Anaerobic energy pathways Slow-twitch, FOG, and fast glycolytic fibers
95-100%	190-200	Anaerobic energy sources Anaerobic energy pathways Slow- and fast-twitch fibers Speed (neuromuscular skill and efficiency)

[a]These figures are only estimates and subject to wide variations between individual athletes.
[b]For a max HR of 200 bpm.

FACTORS AFFECTING HEART RATE MEASUREMENT

Several factors complicate the use of the heart rate as an indicator of training intensity. These factors include the emotions, illness, heat, altitude, the type of exercise involved, and the effects of travel and sleep loss.

Emotions   As you know, the heart rate can speed up when people are emotionally involved in a situation. Situations creating fear and excitement are two examples when the heart rate is not an accurate estimate of effort. Emotionally arousing situations during practice will speed up an athlete's heart rate. Excessive motivation, for example, in a highly competitive practice, can elevate the heart rate, but the effect wears off as the session continues.

Illness   A fever elevates the body temperature and the heart rate, so athletes should not train if they have a fever. After a period of bed rest, the heart rate will also be unusually high. If a youngster has been sick, have him or her return to vigorous training gradually.

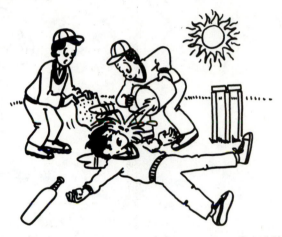

Heat   Exercise in a hot environment raises the heart rate because the body sends blood to the skin as well as to the working muscles as a way of losing heat. When it is unusually hot, by using the heart rate as an indicator of training intensity, you can avoid the dangers of heat stress. The heart rate also climbs when the body becomes dehydrated, so encourage athletes to drink lots of fluids during practice and competition. A failure to drink sufficient water is a common cause of unexpectedly poor athletic performances.

Altitude   During the first week at an altitude above 5,000 feet, the exercise heart rate could be somewhat elevated (no pun intended), but the effect usually goes away within 2 weeks.

Type of Exercise   Certain types of exercise complicate the use of the heart rate as a training guide. Both isometric exercise, where force is exerted against an immovable object, and weight lifting elevate the heart rate beyond that expected for the energy being expended. Also, during work with the arms alone, as in many gymnastic moves, the heart rate is higher than it is for equivalent work performed by the legs. The typical heart rate relationship returns when the arms and legs work together.

Travel and Sleep Loss

Extended travel can elevate the heart rate and hamper performance, especially when you traverse several time zones. Sleep loss also raises the heart rate and decreases the efficiency of aerobic enzymes. Allow extra rest after travel or sleep loss.

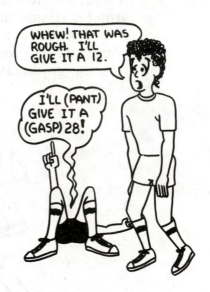

PERCEIVED EXERTION: AN ALTERNATIVE TO CHECKING THE HEART RATE

If the considerations listed above excessively complicate your athletes' training, or if they would rather be freed from the bother of frequent heart rate checks, consider this alternative. The body has thousands of nerves sensing pain, pressure, temperature, and other stimuli. These nerves send messages to the brain, which then computes a composite sense, or perception, of effort. Athletes can learn to read these signals and bypass the need for heart rate checks because *perceived exertion* is usually closely related to heart rate.

To measure perceived exertion, have athletes use the scale (see Table 6.2) developed by Swedish psychologist Gunnar Borg. Instead of taking a heart rate check, athletes simply ask themselves, How does the exercise feel?

During the early days of training use the heart rate *and* the scale. Eventually, the athletes won't need the heart rate; they will be able to properly gauge exercise intensity with their own finely tuned sense of effort. If the training phase calls for exercise at a heart rate of 150 bpm, have your athletes work at the level they judge as hard (rating of 15), and they won't be far off their correct heart rate.

$$Hard = 15 \times 10 = 150 \text{ bpm}$$

Table 6.2
The Perceived Exertion Scale

How does the exercise feel?	Rating
	6
Very, very light	7
	8
Very light	9
	10
Fairly light	11
	12
Somewhat hard	13
	14
Hard	15
	16
Very hard	17
	18
Very, very hard	19
	20

THE TRAINING PYRAMID

Energy fitness training is founded on the basis of the training pyramid illustrated in Figure 6.3. The emphasis coaches place on the different energy fitness components will vary depending on the specific fitness requirements of their sport. In endurance events like marathon running or distance swimming, aerobic and anaerobic threshold training is the major fitness demand. For shorter, faster events like wrestling or baseball, anaerobic and speed training meet the major fitness needs. For all sports, however, progression must be followed to ensure overload and adaptation, and to avoid injury. Let's now review some of the benefits of the four levels of training in the training pyramid.

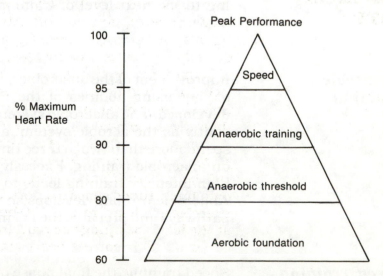

Figure 6.3. The training pyramid.

Aerobic Foundation

In most sports, athletes should first build a solid aerobic foundation. This foundation will prepare the respiratory and circulatory systems, toughen tendons and ligaments, and provide energy for more intense work. Aerobic training also develops the stamina and energy systems of the slow-twitch muscle fibers. Shown in Table 6.3 are general guidelines for aerobic training during the off-season. To use the table you must estimate the amount of *continuous effort* your athletes expend in the sport, then compare this to the training goals.

Table 6.3
Aerobic Foundation Goals

Continuous Effort in Sport	Training Goals[a]
Under 10 s	10-15 mi/wk or 1-2 hr
10 s-2 min	15-20 mi/wk or 2-3 hr
2 min-15 min	20-30 mi/wk or 3-5 hr
15 min-30 min	30-40 mi/wk or 5-7 hr
Over 30 min	Over 40 mi/wk or 7 hr

[a]Runners, football and basketball players, and others who play on foot use miles per week. Swimmers, cyclists, skiers, and other nonrunners use hourly goals.

Anaerobic Threshold

Once a solid aerobic foundation is laid, athletes can proceed to the next level of the pyramid—raising the anaerobic threshold. During this phase, the emphasis is on developing the aerobic capabilities of the FOG fibers. Working at the upper edge of the aerobic work zone raises the anaerobic threshold. In the past, many coaches ignored this phase of energy fitness training, but it is essential preparation for moving to the next level of training—improving the anaerobic system.

Anaerobic Training

Improvement of the anaerobic system should begin when the oxygen-using abilities of the FOG muscle fibers are well developed. The anaerobic system will not improve as significantly as the aerobic system, and it is rarely necessary to spend more than two to three times per week for 6 to 8 weeks on anaerobic training. Excessive emphasis of this difficult, high-intensity training leads to fatigue, illness, and injury. Anaerobic training develops short-term energy sources and pathways and prepares the FG muscle fibers for competition.

Speed Training

Speed training, the final phase of the pyramid, focuses more on neuromuscular development than on improving energy training systems. Speed training is used to sharpen and hone skills before competition. This doesn't mean that all other training should be done slowly; the training pyramid calls for a gradual, systematic increase in speed. However, until the body is ready to handle the stress of intense training, it is sensible to minimize excessive speed work. Well-trained athletes—those who follow a year-round program—are able to handle speed work earlier in the program.

ORGANIZING AN ENERGY TRAINING PROGRAM

How do you begin to organize an energy training program? In order to choose between the many training methods available, you should first consider which methods best fit the needs of your individual athletes.

Selecting Sport-Specific Exercises

Before planning a training program, you must decide what energy sources and pathways are used in the sport and how much attention to give each phase of training. For some sports this decision is easy. For example, in football or baseball, activity rarely lasts more than a few seconds, and therefore relies heavily on the anaerobic energy systems. At the other extreme are sports like cross country skiing and long-distance running that can last over an hour; cleary these depend almost exclusively on the aerobic system. For many sports however, the predominant energy system is less obvious. Depending on the sport, you may also need to distinguish the energy demands of different playing positions. Based on an analysis of the amount of *continuous* effort typically involved in the sport, Figure 6.4 illustrates the relative importance of aerobic and anaerobic energy systems for most sports.

If the continuous involvement is very short as, for example, in football (about 4 seconds per play), your sport is mostly anaerobic. Does that mean you can ignore the aerobic foundation and go directly to anaerobic training? Of course not! In football there are 25 to 30 seconds of rest between bursts of all-out effort. If the players' aerobic fitness is low, as it often is in football, they will not be able to recover between plays and will tire badly in the second and fourth quarters. A strong aerobic foundation also provides the endurance to stand up to long practice sessions; therefore, never ignore the aerobic foundation.

Determining Training Time

Although the relative contribution of aerobic and anaerobic energy during the event is shown in Figure 6.4, how to train or how much time to spend on each phase of training is not. As a general principle, short, intense anaerobic events don't require as much aerobic training as endurance events, and long-endurance events don't need the sprints common to foot-

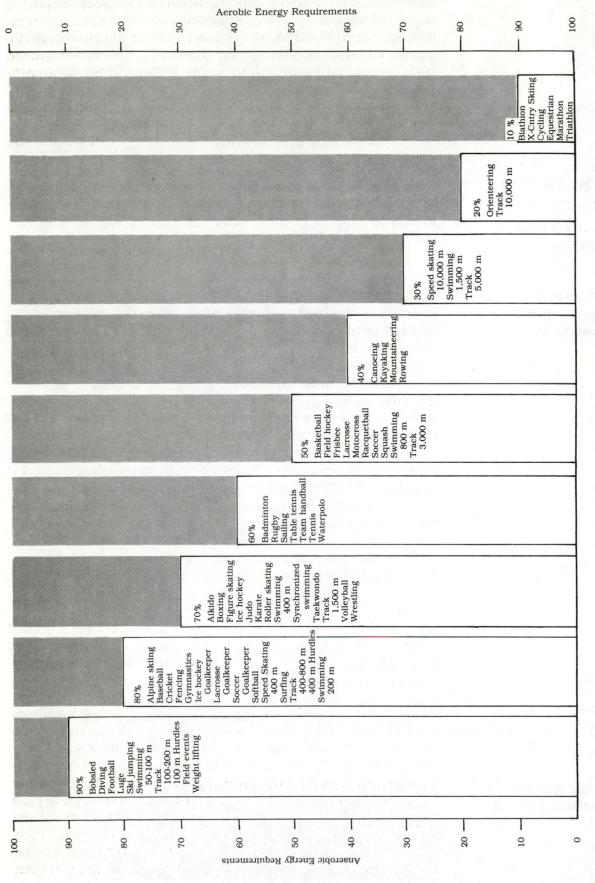

Figure 6.4. Anaerobic and aerobic energy requirements for different sports. *Note.* The following sports have negligible anaerobic energy requirements and can be considered 100% aerobic: archery, boccie, bowling, golf, and the shooting sports.

ball practices. There remain, however, differences of opinion as to the ideal training method for each sport and each individual athlete. Every sport has unique training demands; part of the science of coaching is deciding how much time to devote to each method to have the optimal effect on an athlete's performance. Listed in Table 6.4 are the major energy training methods and their approximate contribution to the development of aerobic and anaerobic energy systems.

By comparing Figure 6.4 and Table 6.4 we can identify the best suited training methods for most sports. This comparison is illustrated in Table 6.5.

Table 6.4
**The Contribution of Different Training Methods
to the Development of Aerobic and Anaerobic Fitness[a]**

Energy Training Methods[b]	Percentage Development of Energy Systems[a]	
	Aerobic (%)	Anaerobic (%)
Continuous training		
Slow paced	95	5
Fast paced	90	10
Hills (if appropriate)	80	20
Fartlek and Repetition training	75	25
Interval training:		
Aerobic: long	70	30
short	60	40
Anaerobic: medium	30	70
short	20	80
Sprints:		
Acceleration	5	95
Hollow sprinting	5	95
Starts and shuttle runs	5	95

[a]These figures are only approximate and depend on how the training method is applied in practice.

[b]Aerobic intervals, fartlek, repetitions, and fast-paced training can be used to train the anaerobic threshold.

Individualizing Training Programs

Remembering to select appropriate training for each *individual* on your team is vital. Some athletes may already have adequate endurance, others may have sufficient power. If you give all athletes the same training, you may provide too much of one thing and not enough of another. The *Coaches Guide to Sport Physiology* provides you with a general training plan based on scientific studies. The art of coaching comes when you adapt that plan to best fit the specific demands of your sport and the needs of individual athletes. Over the years the distinguishing characteristic of great coaches has been their

Table 6.5

Suggested Energy Training Methods for Various Sports and Sport Activities

Sport or Sport Activity	Aerobic							Anaerobic				
	SP	H	F	R	FP	LAI	SAI	MAN	SAN	SPR	ST	SH
Aikido	✓								✓			✓
Archery	✓											✓
Badminton	✓	✓					✓		✓	✓	✓	✓
Baseball	✓	✓	✓	✓	✓			✓	✓	✓	✓	✓
Basketball	✓	✓	✓	✓	✓		✓	✓	✓			
Biathlon	✓	✓	✓	✓		✓						
Bobsled	✓	✓								✓		
Boccie	✓											
Boxing	✓	✓	✓				✓	✓	✓			✓
Bowling	✓											
Canoeing*	✓	✓	✓	✓				✓	✓	✓		✓
Cricket	✓	✓										
Cycling*	✓	✓	✓	✓	✓			✓	✓	✓		✓
Decathlon	✓	✓			✓	✓				✓		
Diving	✓											
Equestrian	✓											
Fencing	✓								✓			
Field hockey	✓	✓	✓	✓			✓	✓	✓	✓		✓
Figure skating*	✓	✓	✓			✓		✓	✓	✓		
Football												
Offensive/defensive linemen	✓	✓	✓		✓		✓		✓	✓	✓	✓
Offensive backs	✓	✓	✓		✓		✓		✓	✓	✓	✓
Receivers	✓	✓	✓		✓		✓		✓	✓	✓	✓
Defensive backs	✓	✓	✓		✓				✓	✓		✓
Kickers/punters	✓	✓	✓		✓				✓	✓		✓
Frisbee	✓	✓							✓	✓		✓
Golf	✓	✓										
Gymnastics	✓								✓		✓	✓
Ice hockey*												
Goalkeeper	✓						✓					
Other positions	✓		✓						✓	✓	✓	✓
Judo	✓						✓		✓	✓		✓

Table 6.5 (Cont.)

Sport	SP	H	F	R	FP	LAI	SAI	MAN	SAN	SPR	ST	SH
Karate	✓			✓			✓	✓	✓	✓	✓	
Kayaking*	✓	✓		✓	✓	✓	✓	✓	✓	✓	✓	
Lacrosse												
Goalkeeper	✓		✓			✓	✓	✓	✓			✓
Other positions	✓	✓	✓	✓	✓	✓	✓	✓	✓	✓	✓	✓
Luge	✓		✓			✓	✓	✓	✓		✓	
Marathon	✓	✓	✓	✓	✓	✓	✓	✓				
Modern pentathlon	✓	✓	✓	✓	✓	✓	✓	✓	✓	✓	✓	
Motocross	✓	✓			✓	✓	✓	✓	✓		✓	
Mountaineering	✓	✓		✓	✓	✓	✓	✓				
Orienteering	✓	✓	✓	✓	✓	✓	✓	✓	✓	✓		✓
Racquetball	✓	✓		✓	✓	✓	✓	✓	✓	✓	✓	
Roller skating*	✓	✓	✓	✓	✓	✓	✓	✓	✓	✓	✓	✓
Rowing*	✓	✓	✓	✓	✓	✓	✓	✓	✓	✓	✓	
Rugby	✓	✓		✓	✓	✓	✓	✓	✓	✓	✓	✓
Sailing	✓	✓			✓	✓	✓	✓				
Shooting sports	✓											
Skiing												
Alpine	✓	✓		✓	✓	✓	✓	✓	✓	✓	✓	✓
Cross-country*	✓	✓	✓	✓	✓	✓	✓	✓	✓	✓	✓	✓
Ski jumping	✓	✓										
Soccer												
Goalkeeper	✓	✓	✓		✓	✓	✓	✓	✓	✓	✓	✓
Other positions	✓	✓		✓	✓	✓	✓	✓	✓	✓	✓	✓
Softball	✓	✓	✓	✓	✓	✓	✓	✓	✓	✓	✓	✓
Speedskating*	✓	✓		✓	✓	✓	✓	✓	✓	✓	✓	
Squash	✓	✓		✓	✓	✓	✓	✓	✓	✓	✓	
Surfing	✓	✓		✓	✓	✓	✓	✓	✓	✓	✓	✓
Swimming*												
50 m all strokes	✓	✓			✓	✓	✓	✓	✓	✓	✓	
100 m all strokes	✓	✓		✓	✓	✓	✓	✓	✓	✓	✓	
200 m all strokes	✓	✓	✓	✓	✓	✓	✓	✓	✓	✓	✓	
400 m all strokes	✓	✓	✓	✓	✓	✓	✓	✓	✓	✓	✓	
800 m all strokes	✓	✓	✓	✓	✓	✓	✓	✓	✓	✓	✓	✓
1,500 m all strokes	✓	✓	✓	✓	✓	✓	✓	✓	✓	✓	✓	

SP — Slow Pace   R — Repetitions   SAI — Short Aerobic Intervals   SPR — Sprints

H — Hills   FP — Fast Pace   MAN — Medium Anaerobic Intervals   ST — Starts

F — Fartlek   LAI — Long Aerobic Intervals   SAN — Short Anaerobic Intervals   SH — Shuttle Runs

*Rather than running, the mode of exercise during the training sessions should be that used in the sport.

Table 6.5 (Cont.)

Sport or Sport Activity	Aerobic							Anaerobic				
	SP	H	F	R	FP	LAI	SAI	MAN	SAN	SPR	ST	SH
Synchronized swimming*	✓					✓		✓				✓
Table tennis	✓						✓					✓
Taekwondo	✓						✓		✓			✓
Team handball	✓	✓					✓	✓	✓	✓	✓	✓
Tennis	✓	✓		✓			✓	✓	✓	✓	✓	✓
Track and field												
100 m	✓	✓					✓		✓	✓	✓	
200 m	✓	✓					✓		✓	✓	✓	✓
400 m	✓	✓					✓	✓	✓	✓	✓	✓
800 m	✓	✓	✓	✓	✓	✓	✓	✓	✓	✓		
1,500 m	✓	✓	✓	✓	✓	✓	✓	✓	✓	✓		
2 mi	✓	✓	✓	✓	✓	✓	✓	✓	✓			
3 mi, 5,000 m	✓	✓	✓	✓	✓	✓	✓	✓	✓	✓		
6 mi, 10,000 m	✓	✓	✓	✓			✓	✓	✓			
100 m hurdles	✓	✓					✓	✓	✓	✓	✓	✓
400 m hurdles	✓	✓					✓		✓	✓	✓	✓
Discus	✓	✓					✓		✓	✓	✓	
High jump	✓	✓					✓		✓	✓	✓	
Javelin	✓	✓					✓		✓	✓	✓	
Long jump	✓	✓					✓		✓	✓	✓	
Pole vault	✓	✓					✓		✓	✓	✓	
Shot put	✓	✓					✓		✓	✓	✓	
Triple jump	✓	✓					✓		✓	✓	✓	
Triathlon	✓	✓	✓	✓	✓	✓	✓	✓	✓	✓	✓	
Volleyball	✓	✓	✓	✓	✓	✓	✓	✓	✓	✓	✓	✓
Waterpolo*	✓			✓	✓		✓		✓	✓	✓	✓
Weight lifting	✓								✓			
Wrestling	✓	✓	✓		✓		✓	✓	✓	✓	✓	

SP — Slow Pace
H — Hills
F — Fartlek
R — Repetitions
FP — Fast Pace
LAI — Long Aerobic Intervals
SAI — Short Aerobic Intervals
MAN — Medium Anaerobic Intervals
SAN — Short Anaerobic Intervals
SPR — Sprints
ST — Starts
SH — Shuttle Runs

*Rather than running, the mode of exercise during the training sessions should be that used in the sport.

ability to match individuals with appropriate training methods. Let's now review the key points of the major energy fitness training methods currently in use.

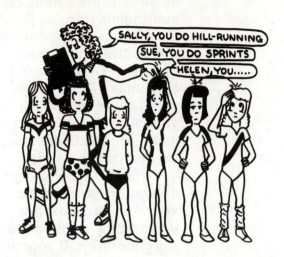

ENERGY TRAINING METHODS

In this section the training methods presented in Table 6.4 are fully described so you can decide the appropriateness of each for your particular sport. Remember, however, that each method is open to modification to more closely meet your individual sport needs.

Sport-Specific Considerations

Specificity of training is essential for the greatest improvements in sport-specific fitness. Running, swimming, skating, skiing, cycling, rowing, and other sport-specific activities can be selected as the principal mode of energy training.

Continuous Training

Exercise that continues without rest intervals is referred to as continuous training. Two types of continuous training are slow-paced and fast-paced training. Slow-paced jogging and lap swimming are currently two of the most popular continuous training methods. Several years ago, many competitive runners turned to long, slow-distance running as the foundation of their training program. Proponents of the method argued that long slow-distance running built up the endurance that provided a foundation for racing speed and that, by avoiding the exhaustion inherent in most other exercise forms, kept training fun.

Slow, continuous training over long distances is the ideal first step for prepubertal, older, and out-of-shape athletes who need to be eased back into shape slowly. For runners, track specialist Dr. Fred Wilt (1968, p. 400-1) recommends distances 2 to 5 times their racing event. I would recommend similar guidelines for athletes in other sports. Athletes should exercise at a comfortable pace that permits normal conversation (approximately 75% of the max HR, 140-160 bpm).

Critics of slow-paced continuous training argue that it does not meet most athletes' specific fitness needs. Regardless of the training mode, long, slow exercise does not simulate the conditions present in a competitive race, whereas fast-paced continuous training does, thereby helping the athlete to better adapt to these conditions. Fast-paced continuous training differs from slow-paced training in training intensity and distance. Your athletes should be working at 80 to 90% of their max HR (at the anaerobic threshold level), for ½ to ¾ the distance required in their sport. This is hard work, so lead your athletes up to fast pace with slow-paced exercise, fartlek, and repetitions. Off-season races and competitions can be used for fast-paced training.

Hills

To increase exercise intensity and add variety to both types of continuous exercise, plan to include some hill training in your program. Exercise over natural rolling terrain or on more demanding uphill sections is an effective method for improving endurance. If your athletes are exposed to uphill sections during competition, hill training should be a vital ingredient in their fitness program.

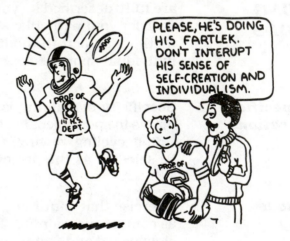

Fartlek

Fartlek, a Swedish word meaning "speed play," is a form of training credited to a Swede named Gosta Holmer. Holmer apparently was seeking a form of running that made use of Sweden's forest paths, simultaneously developing speed and endurance while giving "the feeling of self-creation, of individuality." (*Runner's World*, 1973). The emphasis in fartlek should be on play and on the enjoyment of going fast without excessive pain. Unfortunately, many coaches forget what the word means and turn fartlek into speed *work*. Fartlek involves intervals of faster work followed by easier periods of recovery. Done over natural terrain with a small group of friends, fartlek can indeed be playful. Have the athletes take turns setting a firm pace, but do not allow them to become too competitive.

To train the anaerobic threshold, fast sections should last at least 2 minutes. Explain to your athletes that their mood and the countryside should dictate when to push and when to recover. The faster work on hills helps develop the stamina needed in future workouts. Fartlek works well in running, cross-country skiing, and cycling but can also be used in swimming and other sports. Fartlek is an enjoyable training method that can be modified to emphasize the development of aerobic or anaerobic energy systems. Always remember to select exercises that meet the specific needs of your sport and of your athletes.

Repetitions

Repetitions involve maintaining pace or tempo for intervals of 5 to 12 minutes. Although these workouts can be done on a measured course, many coaches prefer to conduct them away from distance markers, saving the track for shorter interval training. Have your athletes hold a competitive pace on or slightly above the anaerobic threshold for the length of the repetition; then go easy until they recover. Repetitions and other methods of training at or above the anaerobic threshold improve the oxidative, or aerobic, ability of fast-twitch fibers, raise the anaerobic threshold, and prepare the body for fast-paced training.

Depending on how the coach manipulates the variables that affect exercise intensity, the training emphasis can be on improving either aerobic or anaerobic fitness. Repetitions at a pace slower than competitive pace will tend to improve aerobic fitness. Repetitions close to competitive pace are more likely to improve the anaerobic systems. If the training emphasis is on improving anaerobic fitness, and if athletes are performing at close to race speed, the training distance should not exceed 1½ the competitive distance. As an example, shown in Table 6.6 are two sample repetition training programs for a female 1,500-m runner with a best time of 5:00.

Table 6.6
Sample Repetition Training Programs for a 1,500 m Runner[a]

Program	Training Distance	Training Time[b]	Recovery Time[c]	Repetitions
A	1,200 m	83-84 s/400 m 4:09-4:12/1200 m	Heart rate below 120 bpm	2-4
B	2,000 m	85-86 s/400 m 7:05-7:10/2000 m	Heart rate below 120 bpm	1-3

[a]Modified from Wilt (1968).

[b]A best time of 5:00 represents 80 s/400 m. A suitable training pace for 1,200 m is 80 + 3-4 s/400 m, or 4:09-4:12/1,200 m. For 2,000 m the training pace should be increased 5-6 s above the athlete's best time/400 m.

[c]Recovery time depends on the athlete's response to exercise. The athlete should rest until the heartbeat falls below 120 bpm before performing the next repetition.

These two programs are samples of the various ways for organizing repetition training. Follow similar principles to develop repetition programs for your athletes. As you can see, it is easy to design an individualized program to suit each athlete's abilities. With a little experimentation, you'll discover the intensity that seems to produce the greatest benefits. Remember also that the training mode need not be running. Cycling, swimming, rowing, skiing, skating, and many other activities are ideally suited for repetition training.

Interval Training

Interval training involves periods of exercise interspersed with periods of rest. Often, light activity is substituted for total inactivity. By manipulating the following four variables, the training emphasis can be focused on either aerobic or anaerobic energy fitness.

1. Training distance
2. Training intervals
3. Recovery intervals between exercise
4. Repetitions of the exercise

Aerobic Interval Training

Exercise intensity must be controlled to permit your athletes to train the aerobic energy pathways. You want them to improve their ability to use oxygen but not become overfatigued. Although much depends on your athletes and their sport, research suggests that approximately equal training and recovery intervals between 2 to 5 minutes seem to produce the greatest aerobic improvements. Shown in Table 6.7 is a sample aerobic interval program for a high school swimmer. The swim coach who designed this program took the swimmer's best time for each distance (1 min 20 s for 100 yd, and 35 s for 50 yd), then added 10% of this time (8 s and 4 s) to create training intervals of 1 min 38 s and 39 s. Experimentation in the pool verified that by following these intervals, the swimmer was working at approximately 85% of his maximum heart rate—an ideal level to improve aerobic ability. Initially, the coach also allowed the swimmer recovery intervals equal to the training interval but quickly discovered that this was much too easy. Consequently, he reduced the recovery intervals to a level that allowed the swimmer's heart rate to fall to about 120 before repeating the exercise. If you apply these simple principles to your sport, you will be able to design aerobic interval training programs to meet the specific needs of your individual athletes.

Short Aerobic Intervals

To increase the intensity of aerobic interval training, have your athletes work for 15 seconds at a pace above the anaero-

Table 6.7
Sample Aerobic Interval Swimming Program

Set	Training Distance (Yards)	Training Interval (Time)	Recovery Interval (Seconds)	Repetitions
1	100	1 min 38 s	40	4
2	50	39 s	20	8
3	100	1 min 38 s	40	8
4	50	39 s	20	4

bic threshold, followed by easy effort. Twenty to 30 of these "pick-ups" add interest and quality to a longer workout (30 to 60 min). Because the vigorous work interval is so brief, the effort remains essentially aerobic, providing a way to stimulate the aerobic capacities of the fast-twitch muscle fibers. Short aerobic intervals also help to prepare athletes for the faster pace of anaerobic and speed work. Guidelines for aerobic training intervals are shown in Table 6.8.

Anaerobic Interval Training

As illustrated in Figure 6.4, anaerobic energy pathways also contribute to an athlete's fitness for most sports. The intensity of exercise should be closely matched to the demands inherent in competition. A tennis player who typically is involved in 30-second rallies should train intensely for repeated periods approaching 30 seconds.

The maximum duration for any anaerobic training interval is 90 seconds. Beyond this, the anaerobic training effect diminishes as the body turns to the aerobic system to support ongoing activity. Recovery intervals during interval training depend on training time. Shown in Table 6.8 are guidelines for anaerobic training intervals.

Remember, these are general guidelines. Watch the reactions of your athletes closely and, if necessary, be prepared to modify the training intensity.

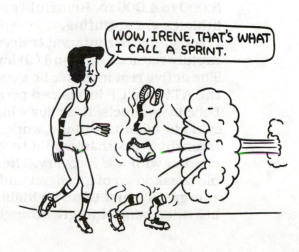

WOW, IRENE, THAT'S WHAT I CALL A SPRINT.

Table 6.8
Guidelines for Aerobic and Anaerobic Interval Training

Types of Intervals and % of Maximum Heart Rate	Training Interval	Recovery Interval[a]	Repetitions	Training Effect
Aerobic				Raises anaerobic threshold
long 80-90%	2-5 min	1:1	4-6	
short 90-95%	15 s	1:1	20-30	
Anaerobic				Improves anaerobic breakdown of glycogen and raises levels of ATP and CP
medium 95-100%	60-90 s	1:2	8-12	
short 100%	30-60 s	1:3	15-20	

[a]Recovery intervals are given in proportion to the training intervals. For example, 1:1 indicates the training and rest intervals should be identical; 1:3 indicates a rest interval 3 times longer than the training interval.

Sprints

All sprint training methods involve periods of maximum effort interspersed with periods of rest. The following methods distinguish themselves by the relationship between rest and exercise. Guidelines for sprint training are shown in Table 6.9.

Interval Sprinting

Interval sprints involve alternate periods of short sprinting followed by easy exercise. Typically, exercise and recovery intervals are of a similar time or distance. For example, a rower might sprint for 15 s then row easily for 15 s, whereas a runner could sprint 150 m and then jog 150 m. Maximum training time should be 10 to 15 min or cover a distance of 3,000 to 4,000 m. Remember to emphasize good form when athletes are sprinting.

As with other interval training techniques, the fast speed rapidly reduces ATP and CP levels and increases lactic acid. The active rest interval, however, provides recovery time for the ATP and CP levels and permits the removal of the metabolic by-products; this allows high-intensity effort to continue. Periods of intermittent work and rest allows more high-intensity work than would be possible following continuous effort or with less recovery. The training improves the anaerobic breakdown of glycogen and raises cellular levels of high-energy ATP and CP. The high-intensity work also loads the heart, causing it to get stronger.

Table 6.9
Guidelines for Sprint Training

Type of Sprints[a]	Training Interval	Recovery Interval[b]	Repetitions	Training Effect
Interval Acceleration Hollow Starts Shuttle runs	10-30 s	1:3	25+	Improves anaerobic break-down of glycogen and raises levels of ATP and CP

[a]All sprints are performed at the maximum heart rate.
[b]Recovery intervals are given in proportion to the training intervals: 1:3 indicates a rest interval 3× longer than the training interval.

Acceleration Sprinting

This is the safest way to improve speed, for the gradual acceleration avoids the most dangerous aspect of sprinting—the rapid start. The training period can be controlled by time or distance. Athletes should gradually accelerate to full speed, hold it for 5 to 15 s or 50 to 100 m (depending on sport-specific requirements), then taper off to an easy pace. The recovery period must be sufficient to enable athletes to perform the next sprint at maximum speed. Acceleration sprints enhance both speed and strength.

This form of training is well adapted to the typical quarter mile or 400-meter track. To do an acceleration sprint, athletes should jog the curve, begin to accelerate as they approach the straight, sprint the straight, and then taper into the curve. With 2 sprints per lap, an athlete will do 8/mi, 24/3 mi. (They'll need a longer rest between each set of 8.) Remember to precede and follow every high-intensity workout with 10 to 15 min of easy effort.

Hollow Sprinting

These are two sprints joined by a hollow period of easy effort. For example, your athletes could sprint 50 m, jog 30 m, sprint 50 m, then walk 50 m to recover before the next training period. This variation adapts well to a country road where athletes can use equally spaced telephone poles to tell them when to sprint. The second sprint should be followed by very easy effort, and the next series started when the athletes are able to sprint in good form. Do not let athletes train with poor form, or they will build bad habits and train the wrong muscle fibers.

Starts

If the sport requires a fast start, have athletes practice starts and sprints from a dead stop. Try to make the drills sport specific; for example, if you coach basketball or tennis, practice sprints on court, running between the lines. Sprinting with the ball or holding the racquet will make drills even more sport related.

Runners, swimmers, skiers, and cyclists need to practice fast starts, regardless of the length of their event. By the late preseason or early competitive season, athletes should be sufficiently conditioned to practice specific speed training, such as running down a slight grade at full speed. Choose a spot that will allow a gradual slowdown. When athletes feel comfortable on a slight grade, choose one a bit steeper. Continue to increase grade and speed until they are running as fast as they can—*safely*. Throughout this training, concentrate on form and on the techniques that seem to help athletes run faster (forward lean, knee lift, push-off, foot strike).

Shuttle Runs

You are probably already familiar with many sport-specific drills that focus on developing speed. Among the most popular for sports requiring fast changes of directions are shuttle runs, also known as line drills. Shuttle runs involve sprinting between marked lines on a field or court. For example, beginning from a starting line, athletes may sprint 10 m to touch a line, turn, sprint back to touch the starting line, turn, sprint 20 m to touch a second line, turn, and follow this sequence for distances up to 50 m. This course is illustrated below:

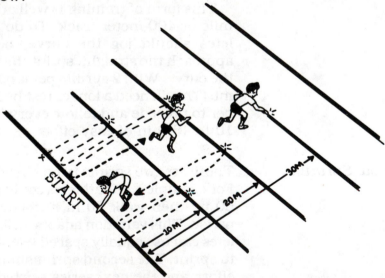

By varying training distances, recovery intervals, and repetitions you can establish an intensity suited to your athlete's needs.

ENERGY FITNESS MAINTENANCE

Regardless of your sport, the energy training program must be founded on the principle of progression. As your athletes progress through the four training stages, do not ignore previous stages in the training pyramid. Aerobic training should be included at every stage in the training session. To maintain previous gains continue with aerobic and anaerobic threshold training during the anaerobic phase and on into the competitive season.

Two aerobic and two anaerobic training sessions per week will maintain the aerobic and anaerobic energy systems. Include competitions in your maintenance plan. During a hectic competitive schedule, less time needs to be devoted to maintenance training. However, many studies have shown that athletes often lose energy fitness as the season progresses, so you should not ignore the need for regular maintenance training. Preoccupation with game plans, strategy, offense, and defense take practice time that was previously available for energy and muscular fitness development. The smart coach ensures that athletes maintain the capabilities they've worked so hard to develop throughout the entire competitive season. In chapter 8 the development of a season plan will be considered in more detail.

SUMMARY

1. Exercise intensity is the most important variable to consider when selecting energy fitness training methods.

2. Intensity can be controlled by monitoring how your athletes' heart rates respond to exercise.

3. Aerobic energy pathways are used if intensity is kept below 85% of the athlete's maximum heart rate.

4. Intensity levels above 85% will improve the anaerobic threshold and anaerobic energy pathways.

5. Illness, heat, and other variables can complicate the use of the heart rate as an indication of exercise intensity. With practice your athletes can learn to gauge intensity by perceiving the required exertion.

6. Energy fitness is founded on the four levels of the training pyramid: aerobic foundation, anaerobic threshold, anaerobic training, and speed training. Although the training focus must depend on sport-specific considerations, training in all sports should follow these progressions.

7. The most appropriate training methods for your sport depends on the relative contributions of aerobic and anaerobic energy systems.

8. The mode of training should be specific to your sport. Cycling, rowing, swimming, skiing, skating, and other exercise forms can be used in addition to running.

9. In addition to sport-specific considerations, also consider individual needs when selecting training methods.

A method for evaluating your athlete's unique physical abilities is the topic of the next chapter.

PART 4
Designing Training Programs

Chapter 7
Athletic Performance Evaluation

To be able to adjust for individual differences, you need to know how athletes differ. Sometimes muscular or aerobic fitness differences are apparent; sometimes they are not. The Athletic Performance Evaluation (APE) is a battery of simple tests you can use to assess your athletes' fitness and performance capabilities. The APE will identify individual differences and will make you more aware of individual variations as you develop and conduct training programs.

The tests in the APE are simple to understand and to administer, and they correlate closely with expensive and time-consuming laboratory tests used to evaluate our nation's top athletes. The APE is an inexpensive tool to help you

- determine current fitness levels,
- identify individual differences,
- assess progress in training,
- spot potential in newcomers, and
- guide athletes to the proper position or event.

As a newcomer to the high school track team, I spent half the season chasing other runners in the quarter- and half-mile events. One day, to avoid a difficult time trial, I asked to work out with the milers. When I came in ahead of the regular distance runners, the coach realized my potential for longer events. The APE test could have identified this ability at the beginning of the season.

The APE test consists of three sections, each containing several tests. First is a general section that tests body type, fat, and muscle fiber type. The second section has tests to evaluate muscular fitness. The final section includes tests of aerobic and anaerobic capacity and of power; these tests will enable you to evaluate energy fitness. Norms for evaluating your athletes' performances are given for each test. Several tests in the APE also appear in the AAHPERD Youth Fitness

Test. For these tests, comprehensive scoring norms for different age groups are available and have been included. Where comprehensive norms are not available, coaches should develop their own scoring tables based on the performance of their athletes.

Will the APE predict success in sport? Although sport scientists have identified attributes and abilities generally associated with success in certain sports (e.g., champion distance runners usually have a high aerobic power), it is *not* possible to use these criteria to predict the outcome of a race or event. Success in sport depends on more than muscles and energy. The APE also has other limitations that must be considered. Differences in maturity, especially during the adolescent period, caution against using these test results for more than a *general* assessment of physical ability. You may also discover that even the physical qualities tested may have little or no relationship to the motor skills needed in the sport you coach. You may find that the athlete who scores poorly on the tests happens to be your best player!

You are advised to view the APE as just one more means of assessing your athletes' *fitness* needs. Use the results to improve those physical qualities that you believe will enhance performance in your sport. Although the APE will help to determine your athletes' fitness and may increase training motivation, do *not* use it to select the team. The stop watch, tape measure, and your own best judgment will do a better job every time.

Illustrated in Table 7.1 is a chart for recording your athletes' scores on the APE. How to evaluate these scores is explained at the end of the chapter.

APE SECTION 1: BODY TYPE, FAT, AND FIBERS

This section of the APE records such basic information as age, height, weight, body fat, and includes a simple test to help you estimate your athletes' muscle fiber type percentage. Information on muscle fiber type percentage could help you discover a budding sprinter or long jumper (fast twitch) or a potential distance runner (slow twitch). As you know, some of the factors related to success in sport are inherited. These factors are body weight, height, physique and fiber type, and each is crucial in certain sports. But, as mentioned earlier, desire and skill can often overcome a handicap in weight or height, so *do not* let this information deter a motivated athlete from pursuing any type of sport interest.

Weight/Height Index

The weight/height index shown in Table 7.2 will help you categorize your athletes' body types as either lean, medium, or heavy. Lean athletes excel in distance events or endurance

Table 7.1
The Athletic Performance Evaluation

Name _____ Age _____

APE Factors	Score	Rating Low	Rating Avg	Rating High	Evaluation
Body type, fat, and fibers					
Weight/height index					
% body fat					
Vertical jump					
Muscular fitness					
Sit and reach					
Pull-ups (males)					
Flex-arm hang (females)					
Push-ups					
Curl-ups					
Stair run					
50-yd dash					
Shuttle run					
Stork stand					
Aerobic fitness					
9 min/1-mi run					
12 min/1.5-mi run					
Anaerobic fitness					
30-s anaerobic capacity					

Table 7.2
Weight/Height Index[a]

Males		Females
Under 2 lb/in.	Lean	Under 1.9 lb/in.
2 to 2.8 lb/in.	Medium	1.9 to 2.5 lb/in.
Over 2.8 lb/in.	Heavy	Over 2.5 lb/in.

[a]Divide the athlete's weight (lb) by height (in.). For example, Juan weighs 140 lb and is 70 in. tall: $140 \div 70 = 2$ lb/in.

sports and low weight classes in wrestling or judo. Medium athletes excel in a wide range of individual and team sports, and heavy athletes are suited for lifting and throwing weights, playing the line in football, and competing in the heavyweight classes in combat sports.

Body Fat and Lean Body Weight

Percentage body fat can be estimated by measuring skinfold thickness (explained in the next section). Too much fat is usually detrimental to performance, while too little can be bad for health. In weight-class sports (e.g., wrestling) and in gymnastics and dance, young men and women often lose too much weight. Use the body fat measure to calculate pounds of fat; then subtract fat weight from total body weight to get the lean body weight. The lean weight consists of muscle, bone, organs, and fluid. A young athlete should *never* weigh less than the lean weight *plus* a certain amount of essential fat. Body fat and lean body weight estimates for one athlete produced the following figures.

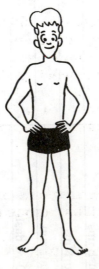

Weight = 150 lb
%fat = 10%
10% × 150 = 15 lb fat
Lean weight = 150 − 15 = 135 lb

Minimum body fat ranges from 5 to 7% for young men to 11 to 13% for young women. Recommendations for minimum body fat measurements for athletes during the different stages of growth and development are given in Table 7.3. Incidentally, boys and girls average 12% and 21% body fat at age 15, and 15% and 25% body fat at 18 to 22 years.

How to Measure Body Fat

Read these general procedures; each part will then be thoroughly explained. With practice you can learn to use skinfold calipers (see Figure 7.1) and the nomogram (see Figure 7.2) to determine percent body fat. If you have not used calipers, take some time to practice using them before giving the APE to your athletes. For more information about measuring body fat, see the *Coaches Guide to Nutrition and Weight Control* (Eisenman & Johnson, 1982).

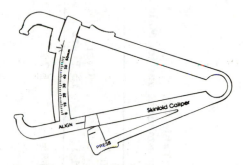

Figure 7.1. Inexpensive skinfold calipers allow accurate estimations of percent body fat. For information on purchasing calipers see Appendix D.

Equipment: Skin calipers, nomogram.

Directions: For males, take skinfold measurements at the chest, abdomen and thigh. For females, measure at the triceps, thigh, and suprailium. Sum the three skinfold measurements and hold a pencil at this figure on the scale provided in Figure 7.2. Take a ruler and draw a line from the skinfold measurement to the athlete's age on the left side of the chart. Read the estimated body fat percentage on the male or female scale.

Directions for Using Skinfold Calipers

1. Take all measurements on right side of body. Look carefully at the illustrations to identify exact measurement locations.
2. Grasp skinfold between thumb and forefinger.

Table 7.3
Minimum Percent of Body Fat Recommendations for Male and Female Athletes

| | Males | | | Females | | |
Sport Category	Under 11 Years	11-15	Over 15 Years	Under 11 Years	11-15	Over 15 Years
High energy/low weight (Wrestling, distance running, gymnastics)	7-9%	6-8%	5-7%	13-15%	12-14%	11-13%
Medium energy/medium weight (Team sports, tennis)	9-11%	8-10%	7-9%	15-17%	14-16%	13-15%
Low energy/high weight (Football, weight lifter, shot, discus)	11-13%	10-12%	9-11%	17-19%	16-18%	15-17%

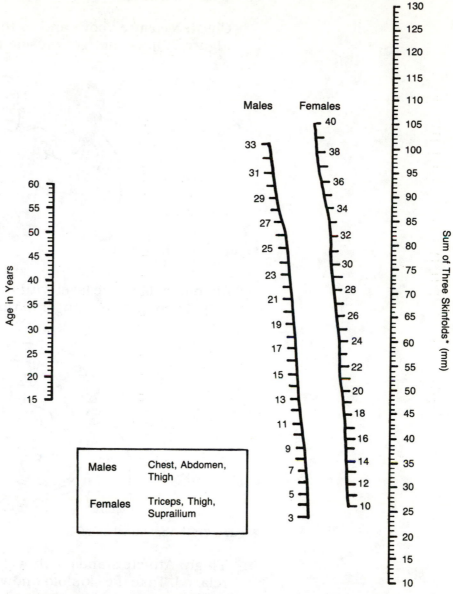

Figure 7.2. Sum of 3 skinfolds. From "A Nomogram for the Estimate of Percent Body Fat from Generalized Equations" by W.B. Baun, M.R. Baun, & P.B. Raven, 1981, *Research Quarterly*, **52**, 382. Copyright 1981 by the American Alliance for Health, Physical Education, Recreation and Dance, 1900 Association Drive, Reston, VA 22091. Reprinted by permission.

3. Place calipers on as far as fold is wide (e.g., if the fold is 10 mm wide, the calipers should be about 10 mm in from the edge of the skin.

4. Squeeze calipers to align lines.

5. Read skinfold in millimeters as you continue to hold the skinfold with your other hand.

6. Remove calipers from fold.

7. Repeat until you get a consistent measure (±2 mm).

To measure males:

Chest: Measure above and to the side of the chest (see Figure 7.3). Do not get muscle caught in the skinfold.

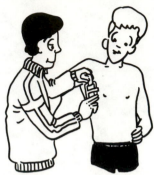

Figure 7.3. Chest skinfold.

Abdomen: Measure level with the umbilicus (see Figure 7.4). Do not put your finger in the athlete's belly button.

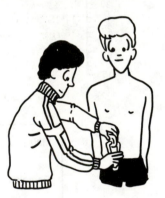

Figure 7.4. Abdominal skinfold.

Thigh: Athlete stands with weight on left leg, right leg relaxed. Take the skinfold midway down the front of the thigh, exactly midway between the knee and hip (see Figure 7.5).

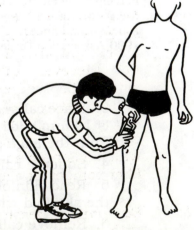

Figure 7.5. Thigh skinfold.

To measure females:

Triceps: Measure at the back of the arm, midway between shoulder and elbow (see Figure 7.6).

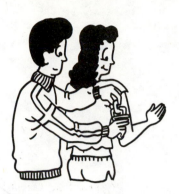

Figure 7.6. Tricep skinfold.

Thigh: As for males.

Suprailium: Above the iliac crest (hip) on the side of the body (see Figure 7.7). Locate top of hip and take the skinfold just above the bone.

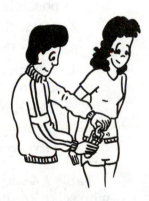

Figure 7.7. Suprailiac skinfold.

Muscle Fiber Type

Fiber types and their relationship to performance in various sports were discussed in chapter 3. It was explained how other factors can offset the influence of slow- or fast-fiber composition. However, athletes may be interested in an estimation of their fiber type composition. One method is to use a needle to take a sample of the fiber type and have this analyzed in a laboratory. This is called a muscle biopsy. A simpler, and certainly less painful method, is to use the following test, which has been shown to correlate with fast-twitch muscle fiber composition (see Figure 7.8).

Evaluating Muscle Fiber Type With the Vertical Jump Test

Equipment: Measuring tape or yard stick taped to the wall with bottom set for the shortest athlete's reach.

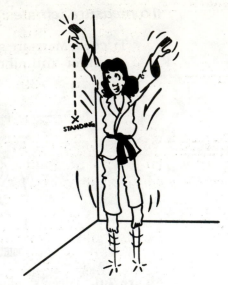

Figure 7.8. Vertical jump test.

Directions:

1. Have the athlete stand beside a wall and touch as high as possible.

2. Mark the spot.

3. Have the athlete chalk the fingers.

4. Instruct the athlete to step back, jump as high as possible, and touch the wall.

5. The difference between the standing reach and the highest point of the jump is the athlete's score.

6. Give each athlete three trials and score the best.

Table 7.4 shows you how to evaluate your test scores. Those who score low have a low percentage of fast-twitch fibers. High scores indicate more fast fibers. Medium scores probably fall

Table 7.4
Relationship Between Vertical Jump Results
and FT Fiber Type Composition

Age and Sex	Low	Average	High
Under 14			
Males	Under 15"	15-20"	Over 20"
Females	Under 8"	8-12"	Over 12"
Over 14			
Males	Under 17"	17-23"	Over 23"
Females	Under 10"	10-15"	Over 15"

in the 50/50 (fast/slow) range. High scores on the aerobic fitness test (1.5-mi run) will help to verify the accuracy of this estimation because high aerobic fitness scores usually indicate a higher percentage of slow-twitch fibers (see aerobic fitness test, page 139).

APE SECTION 2: MUSCULAR FITNESS

This section of the APE evaluates the components of muscular fitness: flexibility, strength, muscular endurance, power, speed, agility, and balance.

Flexibility

Good flexibility improves performance and reduces the risk of injury. Flexibility is crucial in sports like wrestling, gymnastics, swimming, and running. Athletes in all sports will perform better if regular stretching exercises are included in their training programs. The flexibility test illustrated in Figure 7.9 measures the flexibility of your athletes' back and hamstring muscles. You can devise additional tests if flexibility is important in your sport.

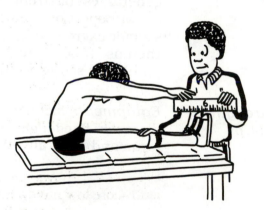

Figure 7.9. Sit and reach test.

How to Measure Flexibility

The sit and reach exercise is a useful test of general flexibility. In Table 7.5 you will find guidelines for evaluating the results of this test.

Table 7.5
Flexibility Ratings From Sit and Reach Test Results

	Low	Average	High
Males	< −3"	−2 to +2"	3+"
Females	< 1"	2 to 4"	5+"

Equipment: Mat or rug and a 12 in. or 18 in. ruler.

Directions:

1. Have athlete sit with legs flat on a mat.

2. Check to make certain that the athlete's legs are flat with toes pointing up.

3. After two warm-up trials, tell the athlete to reach as far as possible and hold this position for several seconds (one hand on top of the other).

4. Hold a ruler so Number 6 is above the athlete's toes.

5. The score is the number of inches (+ or −) reached on the third trial.

Strength

Strength can be determined with expensive laboratory equipment, by lifting weights, or by simple calisthenic exercises like pull-ups (males, see Figure 7.10) or flexed-arm hang (females, see Figure 7.11). Because strength can vary considerably from one muscle group to another, it is important to measure strength as it is used in your sport. Pull-ups are a general test of strength; they may or may not be important in your sport or event. If you can identify a different, sport-specific exercise to test strength (e.g., bench press, leg press), then use this. To evaluate your athletes' performance, compare their scores to the figures in Table 7.6.

Testing Strength Using Pull-Ups (Males)

Equipment: Metal or wooden bar approximately 1½ in. diameter, fixed high enough so that the athlete can hang with arms and legs fully extended and feet off the floor.

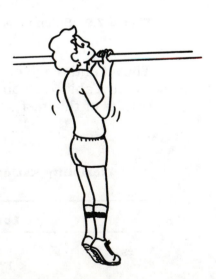

Figure 7.10. Pull-up.

Directions:

1. With palms facing toward the body, have the athletes do as many pull-ups as possible.

2. Do not permit the body to swing during the test or allow athletes to raise their knees or kick their legs.

3. Score the number of pull-ups performed correctly to the nearest whole number.

4. Compare your athletes' scores with the norms in Table 7.6

Table 7.6
Strength Ratings as Estimated
From Number of Pull-Ups Performed[a]

| | | Number of Pull-Ups | |
Age	Low	Average	High
9-10	0	1	6
11	0	2	6
12	0	2	7
13	1	3	8
14	2	4	10
15	3	6	12
16	4	7	12
17+	4	7	13

[a]Data modified from AAHPERD Youth Fitness Test.

Testing Strength Using the Flexed-Arm Hang (Females)

Equipment: Metal or wooden bar approximately 1½ in. diameter, adjusted so that it is approximately level with the athlete's standing height; stopwatch.

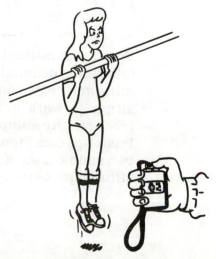

Figure 7.11. Flexed arm hang.

Directions:

1. Athlete holds bar with palms facing toward body and lifts her body off the floor to a position where the chin is above the bar, the elbows are flexed, and the chest is close to the bar.

2. Athlete holds this position as long as possible.

3. Begin the stopwatch as soon as the athlete is in the hanging position.

4. Stop the watch when the chin touches the bar, is tilted backward to avoid the bar, or falls below the bar.

5. Score to the nearest second the time held in the hanging position.

6. Compare your athletes' scores with the norms given in Table 7.7.

Table 7.7
Strength Ratings for Females
as Estimated From Time Held in Flexed-Arm Hang[a]

	Hang Time in Seconds		
Age	Low	Average	High
9-10	3	9	30
11	3	10	30
12	3	9	26
13	3	8	25
14	3	9	28
15	4	9	27
16	3	7	23
17+	3	8	26

[a]Data modified from AAHPERD Youth Fitness Test.

Muscular Endurance

Endurance is the ability to repeat numerous contractions. Certain sports demand high levels of muscular endurance. Swimming and cross-country skiing are typical examples, because although work in these sports never approaches maximal levels, many submaximal contractions must be performed. Push-ups (see Figure 7.12) and curl-ups (see Figure 7.13) are two simple tests of muscular endurance. Coaches should substitute sport-specific tests if these are available.

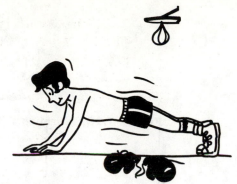

Figure 7.12. Push-ups.

Push-Ups

Equipment: Stopwatch.

Directions:

1. Make sure that the starting position of the hands and feet are the same for all your athletes.

2. Have your athletes perform as many push-ups as possible in 60 seconds.

3. Ensure that the body remains straight as the arms flex.

4. Use Table 7.8 to evaluate your athletes' performance.

Table 7.8
Muscular Endurance Ratings
as Estimated From Number of Push-Ups Performed

Age and Sex	Low	Average	High
Under 14			
Males	Under 15	15-30	Over 30
Females	Under 10	10-20	Over 20
Over 14			
Males	Under 20	20-40	Over 40
Females	Under 10	10-30	Over 30

Curl-Ups

Equipment: Mat or rug and a stopwatch. A padded board with a strap can also be used for testing and training (use as a tilt-board for training).

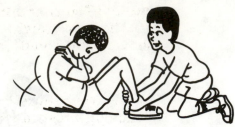

Figure 7.13. Curl-ups.

Directions:

1. Review the correct curl-up technique with your athletes before administering this test.

2. Have each athlete lie on his or her back with knees flexed, heels 12 to 18 in. from buttocks, arms folded across chest with hands on opposite shoulders, and chin tucked to chest.

3. A partner holds the athlete's feet down (see Figure 7.13).

4. On command of "go," the athlete curls up until the elbows touch the legs, then he or she returns to starting position.

5. Ensure that his or her chin remains tucked to the chest.

6. Each curl-up counts as one repetition.

7. The score is the total number of curl-ups completed in 60 seconds. (Repetitions are not counted when hands do not remain on the shoulders or when the elbows come off the chest.)

8. The back should touch the mat before the next curl-up is performed.

9. Evaluate your athletes' performance by referring to Table 7.9.

Table 7.9
Muscular Endurance Ratings
as Estimated From Number of Curl-Ups Performed

Age and Sex	Low	Average	High
Under 14			
Males	Under 15	15-30	Over 30
Females	Under 10	10-20	Over 20
Over 14			
Males	Under 30	30-50	Over 50
Females	Under 25	25-45	Over 45

Caution: Tell your athletes that curl-ups should *not* be done with the legs straight. This can place excessive pressure on the back and could risk injury.

Power

Power, an exciting composite of strength and speed, is tested by moving a resistance as fast as possible. The stair run test and the vertical jump (described earlier) are useful estimates of power.

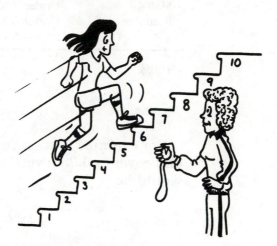

Figure 7.14. Stair run test.

Stair Run Test

Equipment: Stopwatch that records to 100ths of a second; flight of stairs with a 7- or 8-in. rise per step, and at least a 10-ft approach run (see Figure 7.14). *Caution:* Stair running can be dangerous. Warn your athletes of the risks of tripping and falling, and the possible injuries that could occur. Show them how to use their hands to break their fall should they trip on a stair.

Directions:

1. After a demonstration and several slow practice trials, have the athletes run the course—up the stairs two at a time—as fast as possible.

2. Time the run between Steps 2 and 10.

3. Give your athletes three trials, then average their time between the two best trials.

4. Score the results using the following formula; then compare these figures with those outlined in Table 7.10.

$$\text{Power} = \frac{\text{Body wt (lb)} \times \text{Distance (ft)}}{\text{Time (s)}}$$

Table 7.10
Power Rating as Estimated From Stair Run Test Results

Age and Sex	Low	Average	High
Under 14			
Males	Under 600[a]	600-800	Over 800
Females	Under 400	400-600	Over 600
Over 14			
Males	Under 700	700-900	Over 900
Females	Under 500	500-750	Over 750

[a]Ft/lb/s

For example, Dan, a young baseball player, weighs 150 lb and covers a 5.33 ft vertical distance in 1.2 s. His power score would be

$$\frac{150 \times 5.33}{1.2} = 666$$

According to Table 7.10, a power of 666 is lower than average. How important is power to a baseball player? If increased power will improve Dan's performance, the results of the stair test have illustrated the type of training this young athlete needs. You may also find it interesting to compare the times your athletes take for the stair run.

Speed

Speed or quickness is important in most sports. A reliable method of measuring running speed is the 50-yard dash (see Figure 7.15). Although speed comes from muscle fiber type, strength, neuromuscular efficiency, and other factors, it will improve as athletes develop better technique and form and the strength and endurance to sustain that form.

50-Yard Dash

Equipment: 2 stopwatches; 50-yd running course.

Directions:

1. After a good warm-up including stretching and easy running, have athletes run the 50 yd as fast as possible, beginning from a standing start.

2. Introduce a competitive element into the test by testing two athletes at the same time.

3. To start say, "Are you ready?" Then say, "Go!" and simultanteously sweep the arm downward as a signal to the timer who stands on the finish line.

4. Score in seconds to the nearest 10th, and, if time permits, record each athlete's best time from 2 to 3 trials.

5. Compare scores with the norms in Tables 7.11 or 7.12.

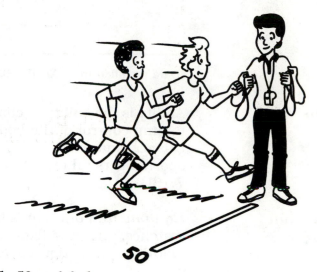

Figure 7.15. 50-yard dash.

Table 7.11
Speed Rating for Males as Estimated
From Time in Seconds on 50-Yard Dash[a]

Age	Low	Average	High
9-10	8.9	8.2	7.5
11	8.6	8.0	7.3
12	8.3	7.8	7.1
13	8.0	7.5	6.7
14	7.7	7.2	6.5
15	7.3	6.9	6.2
16	7.0	6.7	6.2
17+	7.0	6.6	6.1

[a]Data modified from AAHPERD Youth Fitness Test.

Table 7.12
Speed Rating for Females as Estimated
From Time in Seconds on 50-Yard Dash[a]

Age	Low	Average	High
9-10	9.15	8.6	7.7
11	9.0	8.3	7.6
12	8.7	8.1	7.3
13	8.5	8.0	7.1
14	8.3	7.8	7.0
15	8.2	7.8	7.1
16	8.3	7.9	7.2
17+	8.4	7.9	7.1

[a]Data modified from AAHPERD Youth Fitness Test.

Agility

Agility is the ability to change direction quickly while maintaining control of the body. It depends on strength, speed, balance, and coordination. Although agility is specific for each sport, a general test of agility is the shuttle run (see Figure 7.16).

Shuttle Run

Equipment: Four tennis balls and two shoe boxes, two stop watches, and gym floor with two parallel lines—30 ft apart (width of regulation volleyball court).

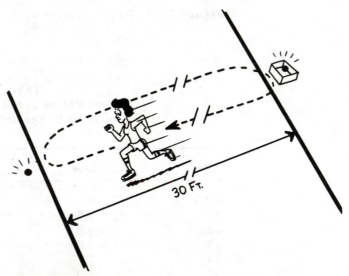

Figure 7.16. Shuttle run.

Directions:

1. Place two balls behind the 30-ft line, facing each athlete.

2. Have the athletes warm up thoroughly, then compete in pairs.

3. Athletes start behind one line; then on the command "Ready" then "Go," they run to the other line, pick one ball, run back to the start, and *place* the ball in the box.

4. Athletes return to get the second ball and finish by placing the ball in the box as they cross the start line.

5. The athlete's score is the time from start to finish (to the nearest 10th of a second).

6. Give each athlete two to three trials to determine the best score.

7. Compare your athletes' scores with the norms in Table 7.13 or 7.14.

Table 7.13
Agility Rating for Males as Estimated
From Time in Seconds on Shuttle Run Test[a]

Age	Low	Average	High
9-10	12.0	11.2	10.3
11	11.5	10.9	10.0
12	11.4	10.7	9.9
13	11.0	10.4	9.6
14	10.7	10.1	9.2
15	10.4	9.9	9.1
16	10.5	9.9	8.9
17+	10.4	9.8	8.9

[a]Data modified from AAHPERD Youth Fitness Test.

Table 7.14
Agility Rating for Females as Estimated
From Time in Seconds on Shuttle Run Test[a]

Age	Low	Average	High
9-10	12.5	11.8	10.6
11	12.1	11.5	10.4
12	12.0	11.4	10.3
13	12.0	11.2	10.2
14	12.0	11.0	10.0
15	11.8	11.0	10.1
16	12.0	11.2	10.3
17+	12.0	11.1	10.0

[a]Data modified from AAHPERD Youth Fitness Test.

Balance

Balance is the ability to maintain equilibrium. Dynamic balance is important in team sports such as basketball, soccer, or football. Static balance is important in sports requiring stationary equilibrium, for example, when a diver stands poised on the edge of the board or a gymnast holds a handstand position. Both balance and agility are sport-specific. They improve with experience in the sport, but they also can improve with participation in a variety of activities. Included here is the stork stand test, which will enable you to measure your athletes' static balance (see Figure 7.17).

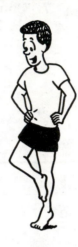

Figure 7.17. Stork stand.

Stork Stand Test

Equipment: Stopwatch.

Directions:

1. Athlete stands on the dominant leg, then places toes of other foot against knee of dominant leg and puts hands on hips.

2. At the commands "Ready" then "Go," athlete raises heel of dominant foot and tries to maintain balance without heel touching floor, foot moving, or hands coming away from hips.

3. Give each athlete three attempts; then compare the best score with the norms in Tables 7.15 and 7.16.

Table 7.15
Static Balance Rating for Males as Estimated
From Time in Seconds Performing the Stork Stand Test

Age	Low	Average	High
Under 10	15	30	45
10-15	25	40	55
Over 15	35	50	65

Table 7.16
Static Balance Rating for Females as Estimated
From Time in Seconds Performing the Stork Stand Test

Age	Low	Average	High
Under 10	10	20	35
10-15	15	30	45
Over 15	25	40	55

APE SECTION 3: ENERGY FITNESS

Aerobic and anaerobic fitness tests can be used to plot progress in a training program, to diagnose individual strengths and weaknesses, and to help select athletes for particular sports.

Aerobic Fitness

Sometimes called cardiorespiratory endurance, or heart-lung fitness, aerobic (with oxygen) fitness is the ability to take in, transport, and utilize oxygen. In events lasting more than 2 minutes (e.g., long-distance swimming, cycling, skiing, and running), aerobic fitness is closely related to performance. In many team sports, the ability to take in and use oxygen helps athletes recover between the intense bursts of activity. Athletes who lack adequate aerobic fitness will tire noticeably as the game wears on. Good aerobic fitness also allows athletes to hold up during long, intense practice sessions.

Aerobic fitness can be measured exactly by a laboratory treadmill test, or it can be estimated using a running test. For athletes under 13, AAHPERD has developed norms for a 1-mile run. For ages 13 and older, a 1.5-mile run is more suitable.

1-Mile Timed Run

Equipment: Running track with known distance markers; stopwatches.

Directions:

1. Pair off athletes and conduct a light warm-up session.
2. Encourage your athletes to run the entire distance, and discourage them from walking.
3. Following the commands "Ready" then "Go," have your athletes run the distance as fast as possible.
4. Have nonrunning partners listen for times as the athlete crosses the finish line.
5. Norms for boys and girls for the tests are presented in Tables 7.17-7.18.

Table 7.17
Aerobic Fitness Rating for Males
as Estimated From Time in Minutes and Seconds
Performing the 1-Mile Run[a]

Age	Low	Average	High
10	10:25	9:07	6:52
11	10:02	8:44	6:31
12	9:39	8:21	6:06

[a]Data modified from AAHPERD Youth Fitness Test and Texas Physical Fitness-Motor Ability Test.

Table 7.18
Aerobic Fitness Rating for Females
as Estimated From Time in Minutes and Seconds
Performing the 1-Mile Run[a]

Age	Low	Average	High
10	11:42	10:29	8:22
11	11:11	9:58	7:51
12	10:37	9:24	7:17

[a]Data modified from AAHPERD Youth Fitness Test and Texas Physical Fitness-Motor Ability Test.

1.5 Mile Timed Run   Follow identical administrative procedures as explained for the previous tests. Use these tests for athletes ages 13 and older, and compare scores to the norms presented in Table 7.19. An alternative method for estimating your athletes' aerobic fitness is shown in Figure 7.18, which then uses Table 7.20 to evaluate the results.

Table 7.19
Aerobic Fitness Rating for Males and Females
as Estimated From Time in Minutes and Seconds
Performing the 1.5-Mile Run[a]

Age	Low	Average	High
Males 13+	12:39	11:29	9:29
Females 13+	18:50	16:57	13:38

[a]Data modified from AAHPERD Youth Fitness Test and Texas Physical Fitness-Motor Ability Test.

Table 7.20
Aerobic Fitness Rating for Males and Females
as Estimated From the Oxygen Cost of Running 1.5 Miles

	Aerobic Fitness[a]			
	Low	**Average**	**High**	**Very High**
Males	Under 45	45-55	55-65	Over 65
Females	Under 40	40-50	50-60	Over 60

[a]Score is in milliliters of oxygen per kilogram of body weight per minute (ml/kg/min).

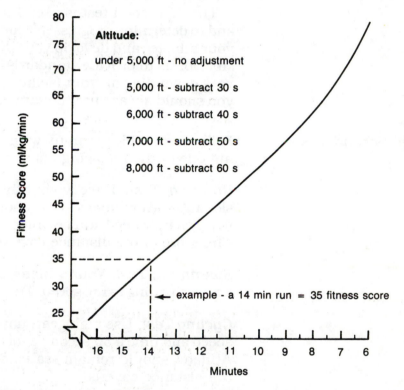

Figure 7.18. Aerobic fitness evaluation as estimated from the oxygen cost of running 1.5 miles. (Data modified from Balke, 1963; Cooper, 1970; Sharkey, 1977.)

Successful distance athletes tend to score in the very high category; soccer players should score high, and even football players should be in the medium category. Athletes who score low in aerobic fitness are probably out of shape.

Anaerobic Power and Capacity

Anaerobic means without oxygen; it describes exercise that is so intense that oxygen intake can't keep pace. In the lab, anaerobic ability is determined by taking muscle biopsies, or lactic acid measurements.

Anaerobic Power

Anaerobic power is a combination of short-term energy and muscle power. Short-term anaerobic power can be estimated with the stair run test described earlier in the Power section of the APE. This test correlates highly with success in power sports such as football, wrestling, and judo, and with several of the throwing and jumping events in track.

Anaerobic Capacity

Longer duration anaerobic capacity can be inferred from a 30-second all-out effort, for example, in running, swimming, or cycling. The ability to sustain a fast pace indicates a higher lactic acid capacity. This ability is needed in short, intense, sustained events (220 yd to a mile in track, 100- to 500-m swims), and in longer events that include periods of anaerobic work such as cross-country skiing and cycling.

The 30-second test is useful to assess anaerobic capacity and to determine progress in training. Compare scores among your athletes and develop your own set of norms. It's not possible for us to provide standards because test conditions will vary depending on your facility. Because of these variations, you should always use the same course when giving the test.

30-Second Test

Follow a suitable warm-up with a 5-min rest before conducting one of the following tests:

Running Test. Have your athletes run up a moderately sloping road or fairway. They should use a 10-yd running start to reach full speed and be timed after a 30-second all-out run. The score is the distance covered in 30 seconds.

Swimming Test. Your athletes should swim 30 seconds after accelerating to full speed. The score is the distance covered.

Cycling Test. Use high gear; have your athletes pedal to full speed and time a 30-second effort on a gradually sloping road. Athletes should remain seated during the test. The score is the distance covered.

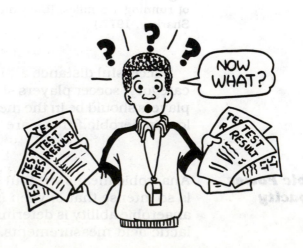

HOW TO USE THE APE

To use the APE, you should record the scores of your athletes on a chart similar to the one illustrated in Table 7.1. Careful examination of these results will help you to identify the strengths and weaknesses of each athlete and to develop training programs suited to each athlete's specific needs. As an example of this process, Table 7.21 illustrates data obtained on the APE test for a 16-year-old midfield soccer player. The coaches evaluation follows:

Table 7.21
The Athletic Performance Evaluation

Name _Eric_   Age _16_

APE Factors	Score	Low	Rating Avg	High	Evaluation
Body type, fat, and fibers					
Weight/height index	130 lb/70 in = 1.86				Lean
% body fat	8 %				Lean
Vertical jump	17 in		✓		needs work
Muscular fitness					
Sit and reach	+2		✓		
Pull-ups (males)	6		✓		
Flex-arm hang (females)					
Push-ups	35		✓		
Curl-ups	53				
Stair run	690		✓		needs work
50-yd dash	5.2		✓		needs work
Shuttle run	9.5		✓		needs work
Stork stand	> 30 sec				
Aerobic fitness					
9 min/1-mi run					
12 min/1.5-mi run	50		✓		needs work
Anaerobic fitness					
30-s anaerobic capacity	Average				needs work

APE Evaluation

Eric's weight/height index and body fat evaluation indicate that he is lean; this is appropriate for soccer. His flexibility is adequate but his vertical jump (17 in.) is low for a sport where players must leap high to head the ball. Consequently, Eric's coach makes a note to include specific leg strength and power training during the off-season and preseason. Incidentally, the low vertical jump suggests that he probably has less than 50% fast-twitch muscle fibers.

Regarding endurance, Eric's trunk endurance (curl-ups) is high. His coach expected this but was surprised to discover that Eric's leg power is low. This confirmed the need for off-season training that should also improve his time in the 50-yd dash. Eric's agility needs to be better for soccer, so the coach schedules more agility drills, including some with the ball as the season approaches.

In terms of energy fitness we've already seen that Eric is somewhat low in power (stair run). The coach's favorite test, the 30-second run up the hill behind the school, indicates that Eric is only average among his teamates in anaerobic capacity. Because a soccer halfback needs to be able to sustain bursts of speed, the coach will include some 30- to 60-second intervals to improve anaerobic capacity in the weeks leading up to the start of the season. Finally, and most important for a midfield player, Eric's aerobic fitness could be improved. His position calls for almost continuous movement, and aerobic fitness forms the foundation for such endurance. Eric will be encouraged to include more distance work in the off-season training program. When practice begins the coach will schedule time for preseason training of the anaerobic threshold. Sustained speed is often the difference between a good athlete and a great one.

SUMMARY

1. The Athletic Performance Evaluation (APE) is a battery of simple physical tests coaches can use to assess the fitness and performance capabilities of their athletes.

2. The APE can be used to guide and motivate training and to help young athletes select a sport or position ideally suited to their physical characteristics.

3. The APE is also useful for monitoring an athlete's progress during the season or between seasons.

4. Coaches should *not* use the tests in the APE to select their team. Young athletes must be given time to grow and develop, to try new skills, to experience a regular training routine, to learn the importance of proper rest and nutrition, and to know what is needed to put it all together on the day of the game. Coaches should remember that not even the most sophisticated computerized laboratory profile can predict the outcome of a sports contest. Desire, determination, and a little extra effort will often triumph over ability.

Chapter 8
Training Program Development

In previous chapters, differences between muscle fibers, energy systems, and other physiological principles were explained. This chapter takes the theory and puts it into practice by providing step-by-step guidelines to the formulation of seasonal training programs for muscular and energy fitness. The various phases of the year-round training program will be considered first.

SEASONAL TRAINING

As mentioned earlier, the training focus for young, preadolescent athletes should be on fun and development. Many athletes enjoy the variety of changing sports from season to season and are not interested in specializing in just one sport. For these athletes, a year-round training program based on the requirements of one sport is inappropriate. If you only have your athletes for 15 weeks of the year, you must adapt your training plan to fit this schedule.

As young athletes grow more proficient, however, some will want to concentrate on just one sport. When this occurs, coaches should be prepared to offer sound advice on developing a year-round training program to develop sport-specific physical abilities. This doesn't mean that athletes can't compete in other sports or play for relaxation. It just means that training decisions must be made to suit your athletes' primary sport. Consider, for example, Mike, an up-and-coming young wrestler. He trains seriously during the fall, competes in the winter, tapers off a bit in the spring, and then competes in summer regional contests. Between seasons he runs for fun and fitness. He lifts weights in the off-season but doesn't let the training interfere with his love of canoeing and backpacking.

Laura is a cross-country ski racer in the winter and a cyclist in the spring and summer. The sports complement each other, so she seldom has a conflict. When the competitive cycling season is over, she begins off-snow training for skiing. Between seasons, Laura runs a few road races to ensure intensity in her training. Finally, she works on upper body strength and endurance training in the fall to prepare for the first snowfall.

Of course, as athletes develop more serious interest in excelling in a sport, training must become more specialized, and participation in other sports may have to be sacrificed. This can be a stressful period, and your athletes will be relying on you for advice and support. It may help to remind them that they should *not* be striving to meet goals established by their parents, coaches, or friends. Excellence in sport comes from an inner motivation combined with good coaching advice. As you review the four phases of the year-round training program, consider how to best apply the recommendations to your sport and to your unique group of athletes.

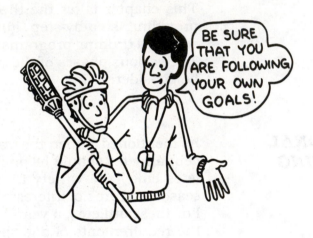

BE SURE THAT YOU ARE FOLLOWING YOUR OWN GOALS!

Off-Season Training

The main purpose of off-season training is usually to keep athletes involved in moderate activity, thereby avoiding the excessive weight gains that hinder participation during strenuous activity. Inactive athletes will also tend to lose the developmental gains achieved in the previous playing season.

Muscular fitness training should focus on improving strength and power in the muscle groups used in your sport and also on eliminating individual deficiences of which you are aware from personal observation or from an evaluation test such as the APE. Three training sessions per week are usually sufficient for off-season muscular fitness gains.

Energy fitness training for most sports should concentrate on developing a solid aerobic foundation. Remember that aerobic fitness forms the foundation of the training pyramid and is the springboard for more intense activity. Typical activities might include slow and fast continuous exercise, fartlek, and easy-paced interval training. A variety of aerobic activities will add interest and variety to off-season training. Two or three energy fitness training sessions per week are probably sufficient in the off-season. Because of the low intensity, both muscular fitness and energy fitness training programs can be done on the same days. A sample schedule follows:

	Muscular Fitness	*Energy Fitness*
Sun		
Mon	Weight training	Continuous slow exercise
Tues		
Wed	Weight training	Fartlek
Thurs		
Fri	Weight training	Continuous slow exercise
Sat		

These suggestions are open to modifications to suit your athletes' off-season schedules and sport-specific fitness demands. This is also an ideal time to encourage participation in other sport or recreational activities and to practice sport-specific skills.

Physiological Benefits of Off-Season Training

Several weeks of strength and power training create a solid foundation for further muscular fitness gains. Off-season energy training develops the oxygen-using enzymes of the slow-twitch fibers. As training continues, the muscles gain ability to use oxygen for fat metabolism. Other benefits of this training are improved respiration and circulation. The heart can slow its rate, and more blood is pumped with each beat. The blood volume is increased and the body's store of hemoglobin is improved. Capillaries serving the muscles become more numerous, further enhancing oxygen delivery to the muscles. Other changes include improved hormonal function and stronger bones, ligaments, and tendons.

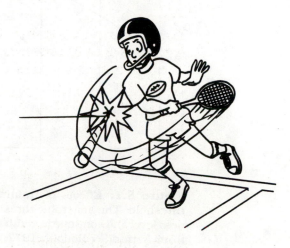

Preseason Training

The preseason training phase for most sports begins 8 to 10 weeks prior to the start of the competitive season. Training intensity for both muscular and energy fitness should increase during this period. In addition to improving muscular strength and power, muscular endurance training should be introduced if this is a key quality in your sport.

An increase in the intensity of energy training will recruit and train FOG muscles fibers. Games, matches, and races are often won with speed, and that requires well-trained fast-twitch fibers. The average athlete has about 35% FOG fibers. It would be foolish to ignore the possible contributions of these fibers to performance. Preseason training should include a variety of the faster paced energy training methods (see Table 6.4 for a list of training methods). These methods will overload the oxidative capabilities of the FOG fibers and thereby raise the anaerobic threshold. As training progresses and more FOG fibers gain endurance, athletes will be able to sustain a faster pace for a longer distance or duration.

Physiological Benefits of Preseason Training

The higher intensity training recruits FOG fibers, overloads their aerobic, or oxygen-using systems, and raises the anaerobic threshold. As you can see from Figure 8.1, in the initial months athletes are only able to work at 50 to 60% of their aerobic fitness capacity before hitting the anaerobic threshold level. However, as conditioning improves, athletes can work at up to or above 80% of their aerobic fitness capacity before the anaerobic threshold becomes a limiting factor. This improvement is of critical importance in all aerobically focused sports.

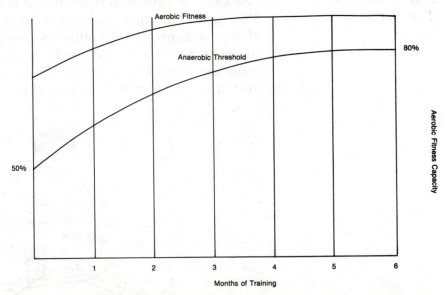

Figure 8.1. Effects of training on aerobic fitness and the anaerobic threshold. The anaerobic threshold can rise above 80% of the aerobic fitness level and continue to climb long after aerobic fitness plateaus. (Adapted from Astrand & Rodahl, 1977; Sharkey, 1977.)

Research shows that best results occur when training is at or is slightly above the anaerobic threshold. For most athletes this means training at 85 to 90% of their maximum HR, gauging their threshold by respiration or heartbeat or by the perceived exertion chart (see page 97). Athletes should work at a perceived exertion level slightly above very hard— approximately 17, or 170 bpm, and sustain work on or slightly above the anaerobic threshold for more than 2 minutes to ensure adequate involvement of the aerobic energy pathways.

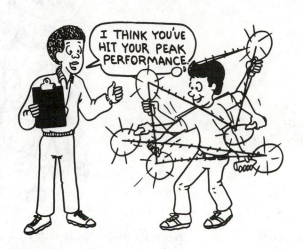

Early Season Training

The early season is the time to work on sport-specific power and speed training. High-intensity training sessions should be planned to build up to important competitive dates. For many sports, especially team games, planning for a competitive peak is complicated by the fact that athletes must perform well over a period of several weeks. Weekly training must be designed to prepare athletes to regularly peak on game days. In other sports, track and field, for example, athletes typically train to peak for prestigious competitions. Their build-up is gradual, and early season competitions are used for training purposes. How does your sport compare to these examples? These differences must be considered as you plan your athletes' training programs.

If anaerobic fitness is critical to your sport, 6 to 8 weeks of high-intensity anaerobic workouts, 2 to 3 times each week is probably sufficient to enable your athletes to meet their anaerobic training goals. If during this time your athletes are involved in early competitions, you should count these as high-intensity sessions. Interval training and a selection of the various sprint training methods will ensure training is focused on anaerobic development.

*Physiological
Benefits of
Early Season
Training*

Anaerobic training will improve the capability of muscle fibers to produce energy from muscle glycogen. The more intense sprint-training methods develop additional short-term (ATP & CP) energy sources and increase speed by improving neuromuscular coordination.

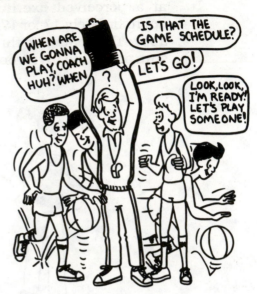

**Peak Season
Training Programs**

As you approach the height of the competitive season, muscular and energy fitness training typically culminate in an emphasis on speed. High-speed training tops off the muscles' supply of high-energy ATP and CP. Speed training also prepares the body for the intensity and quality of late season competition. Skills must be practiced at a high speed to simulate competitive conditions. So speed training not only readies the energy and skills athletes will need, it also may help them perform just a bit faster.

During the competitive season, athletes in most sports must concentrate on high-speed/low-resistance movements and sprints. In addition to using weights and variable resistance training devices, specialized sport-specific speed training should also be included in training. For example, a baseball outfielder noted for a poor arm could use weights in the off-season, power training in the preseason, and all-out speed training as the season gets under way. Using pulley weights in the throwing motion will build strength; then weighted balls will build power, and isokinetic training will improve the throwing motion. All-out throwing for distance or throwing as hard as possible against a wall could provide additional speed.

*Peak Season Fitness
Maintenance*

As the competitive schedule becomes more intense, the bulk of training time will probably be spent on skill refinement. However, even regular competition and competitive practice drills are unlikely to be sufficient to maintain the muscular and energy fitness gains obtained in the previous seasonal training phases. If athletes are not involved in regular competition, or if muscular fitness declines, you should organize a program for maintaining fitness. Several studies have shown that many athletes lose strength, endurance, power, and other fitness components as the season progresses.

The key to peak season maintenance programs is to select sufficient but not excessive exercise to maintain your athletes' competitive peak. This will vary from athlete to athlete and from sport to sport. It is clear, however, that one to two fitness sessions each week are sufficient to maintain most athletes' fitness level. You do *not* want your athletes to enter competition exhausted from participating in your peak season fitness sessions. If competitive drills or activities that simulate typical competitive conditions are integrated into training, these may substitute for fitness sessions. A summary of recommended procedures for developing seasonal programs is outlined in Table 8.1.

DEVELOPING INDIVIDUAL-IZED TRAINING PROGRAMS FOR DIFFERENT SPORTS

To help you design a training program suited for your athletes, sports have been grouped according to their muscular and energy fitness requirements. Table 8.2 presents an alphabetical listing of most sports along with their fitness demands. In Table 8.3 these same sports are grouped with others of similar muscular or energy demands. The designations (low, medium, high) indicate the amount of *time* that must be spent in the development of either muscular or energy fitness. Sports in the low category require little training time for that component of fitness; those in the high category require a great deal of time. Often, sports in the low category (e.g., golf) do not require much fitness training time, but they involve considerable practice to develop, fine tune, and maintain the necessary skills.

Muscular Fitness Training

Each sport has its own particular muscular fitness needs: These depend on the movements and muscle groups involved. Once you have identified these needs, you must select training exercises appropriate for the age, skill, and experience of your individual athletes. The final step is to integrate these exercises into a seasonal training plan. The training principles and methods outlined in chapters 3 and 4 are your guide to the day-to-day conduct of the program.

Energy Fitness Training

The time spent for energy fitness training depends on the dominant energy fitness needs of the sport or position. The information in Table 8.3 will help you make this decision. Those sports categorized as low may only require 20 to 30

**Table 8.1
Seasonal Training Outline**

Off-Season	Preseason	Early Season	Peak Season
Muscular fitness training to improve strength and power in sport-specific muscle groups (8 weeks, 3x/week).	Muscular fitness training of increasing intensity for strength, power, and endurance (8 to 10 weeks, 3x/week).	Muscular and energy fitness sessions of high-intensity, focusing on sport-specific power and speed; frequency depends on competitive schedule (1 to 3x/week).	Speed is the emphasis in fast sports. Use high-speed/low-resistance movements and sprints (1 to 2 sessions/week).
Energy fitness training to improve aerobic ability; low-intensity, continuous exercise, fartlek, and interval training (8 weeks, 2x/week).	High-intensity energy fitness training, including intervals and sprints (8 to 10 weeks, 3x/week).	Anaerobic fitness is critical; high-intensity sessions (6 to 8 weeks, 2 to 3x/week).	Use competitive skill drills in training.
Participation in other sport and recreational activities.	Strategy, technique, and skill practice.	Sport-specific skills, strategies, and competitive drills.	Regular competition substitutes for fitness sessions.
Practice sport-specific skills. Keep body fat low.			

Table 8.2
Muscular and Energy Fitness Training
Requirements for Different Sports

Sport	Muscular Fitness	Energy Fitness
Aikido	Medium	Medium
Archery	Low	Low
Badminton	Medium	Medium
Baseball	Medium	Low
Basketball	Medium	Medium
Biathlon	Medium	High
Bobsled	Medium	Low
Boccie	Low	Low
Boxing	High	Medium
Bowling	Low	Low
Canoeing	Medium	High
Cricket	Medium	Low
Cycling	Medium	High
Decathlon	High	Medium
Diving	High	Low
Equestrian	Low	Low
Fencing	Medium	Low
Field hockey	Medium	Medium
Figure skating	High	Medium
Football		
Offensive/defensive linemen	High	Low
Offensive backs	Medium	Medium
Receivers	Medium	Medium
Defensive backs	Medium	Medium
Kickers/punters	Medium	Low
Frisbee	Medium	Medium
Golf	Low	Low
Gymnastics	High	Medium
Ice hockey		
Goalkeeper	Medium	Low
Other positions	Medium	Medium
Judo	Medium	Medium
Karate	Medium	Medium
Kayaking	Medium	High
Lacrosse		
Goalkeeper	Medium	Low
Other positions	Medium	Medium
Luge	Medium	Low
Modern pentathlon	High	Medium
Motocross	Medium	Medium
Mountaineering	Medium	High
Orienteering	Medium	High
Racquetball	Medium	Medium
Roller skating	Medium	Medium
Rowing	Medium	High
Rugby	Medium	Medium
Sailing	Medium	Low
Shooting sports	Low	Low

Table 8.2 (cont.)

Sport	Muscular Fitness	Energy Fitness
Skiing		
Alpine	Medium	Medium
Cross-country	Medium	High
Ski jumping	Medium	Low
Soccer		
Goalkeeper	Medium	Low
Other positions	Medium	Medium
Softball	Medium	Low
Speedskating	Medium	Medium
Squash	Medium	Medium
Surfing	Medium	Medium
Swimming		
50 m all strokes	Medium	Medium
100 m all strokes	Medium	Medium
200 m all strokes	Medium	High
400 m all strokes	Medium	High
1,500 m all strokes	Medium	High
Synchronized swimming	Medium	Medium
Table tennis	Medium	Medium
Taekwondo	Medium	Medium
Team handball	Medium	Medium
Tennis	Medium	Medium
Track and field		
100 m	Medium	Medium
200 m	Medium	Medium
400 m	Medium	Medium
800 m	Medium	High
1,500 m	Medium	High
2 mi	Medium	High
3 mi/5,000 m	Medium	High
6 mi/10,000 m	Medium	High
100 m hurdles	High	Medium
400 m hurdles	High	Medium
Marathon	Medium	High
Discus	High	Low
High jump	High	Low
Javelin	Medium	Low
Long jump	Medium	Medium
Pole vault	High	Medium
Shot put	High	Low
Triple jump	Medium	Medium
Triathlon	Medium	High
Volleyball	Medium	Medium
Water polo	Medium	High
Weight lifting	High	Low
Wrestling	High	Medium

Table 8.3
Muscular and Energy Fitness Groups for Different Sports

Muscular Fitness	Energy Fitness	Sport or Event
Low	Low	Archery, boccie, bowling, equestrian, golf, shooting sports
Medium	Low	Baseball, bobsled, cricket, fencing, football (kicker/punter), ice hockey goalkeeper, javelin, lacrosse goalkeeper, luge, sailing, ski jumping, soccer goalkeeper, softball
High	Low	Discus, diving, football (linemen), high jump, shot, weight lifting
Medium	Medium	Aikido, badminton, basketball, football (offensive and defensive backs, receivers), field hockey, frisbee, ice hockey, judo, karate, lacrosse, long jump, motocross, racquetball, roller skating, rugby, skiing (alpine), soccer, speed skating, sprints, squash, surfing, swimming (sprints), synchronized swimming, table tennis, taekwondo, team handball, tennis, triple jump, volleyball
High	Medium	Boxing, decathlon, figure skating, gymnastics, hurdles (100 m/400 m), modern pentathlon, pole vault, wrestling
Medium	High	Biathlon, canoeing, cycling, distance running, kayaking, mountaineering, orienteering, rowing, skiing (cross-country), swimming (above 200 m), triathlon, water polo

minutes of energy fitness training a day. High-energy sports, such as swimming or cycling, may require 1 to 2 hours of training daily. You will also need to balance out the proportion of time to be devoted to aerobic and anaerobic training.

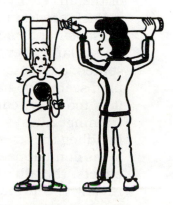

Individual differences in muscular and energy fitness can be determined with the help of fitness tests such as the Athletic Performance Evaluation (APE) together with your own personal observations. Do not waste your athletes' time by having them spend more time on fitness training than is appropriate for their sport. I've met many swimmers and skiers who have far more strength than members of the U.S. Olympic Squads but who cannot compete at the same level. If strength, endurance, or any other fitness component is at an adequate level, direct your athletes to concentrate on other phases of training such as improving their technique and psychological skills. Remember, also, to consider individual differences in age, experience, and development. Training guidelines for young prepubertal children were given in chapter 2. Exceeding recommended exercise intensities with youngsters spoils the pleasure of sport participation and may cause physical harm.

Sample Sport-Specific Training Plans

Sample seasonal training programs appropriate for the muscular and energy fitness demands for a sport in each of these fitness groups follow. These programs serve as examples to help you develop your own program. Use them as a guide to program development, but don't be afraid to add your own ideas as you grow in knowledge and experience. The sample plans are necessarily general and lack many of the specifics you must add to make them practically useful. Be willing to supplement these ideas with the advice of respected coaches in your sport. Try to stay current with the latest training techniques by regularly consulting coaching books and attending coaching clinics. Remember that for all sports, neither research findings nor the observations of successful coaches point to a single most effective system of training. The sample programs in this chapter are models of a developmental process to which you must adapt to meet the specific needs of the athletes you coach.

Each program begins with a brief discussion of the major muscular and energy fitness needs. Then a plan that outlines muscular and energy fitness training for each season is presented. Remember, that these plans are only examples. If the plan seems too hard for your athletes, make adjustments; if it is too easy, carefully increase the quality or quantity of training. Always stay aware of how your young athletes are handling the stress. Sometimes the effects of several hard sessions don't appear immediately, and by the time you see the effects, the athletes may already be worn down. Regularly review the principles of training and utilize the ideas for preventing overtraining presented in chapter 9.

SAMPLE PROGRAM FOR LOW-MUSCULAR, LOW-ENERGY TRAINING: GOLF

This program is designed for golf where skill demands are high and muscular and energy demands are low. Improvements in strength or endurance won't necessarily improve golf skills, but they may allow an athlete to maintain those skills throughout a long match or tournament. And they could help add length to your golfer's game.

Identifying Fitness Needs

Muscular Fitness

The muscular fitness demands in golf are generally low; however, golfers may benefit from exercises to develop muscle groups in the upper body used during the swing. Although their legs are less important, golfers must be capable of walking long distances, often supporting a full set of clubs. Flexibility in the shoulders and lower back is especially important, and twisting exercises for the trunk and wrists are ideal for golfers. Listed below are the principle muscle groups and weight-training exercises recommended earlier (in Table 4.3) for golfers.

Muscle Groups	Weight-Training Exercise
Lower and upper back, upper legs	Half squat
Upper and lower arm	Arm curl
Upper arm	Incline press
Shoulder, upper arms	Military press
Shoulder, upper and lower	Parallel bar dips
Shoulder	Upright rowing
Chest, upper arms	Bench press
Trunk, shoulder girdle	Power clean
Trunk, shoulder girdle	Swing with weighted club
Abdomen	Bent-knee sit-ups
Forearm	Reverse wrist curl
Forearm	Wrist curl or wrist roller

A selection of 8 to 10 of these exercises will be sufficient for a weight training program for young golfers. From time to time you may wish to vary exercises to stimulate interest or to meet specific individual needs. For example, if you notice that one of your golfers has problems gripping the club, the problem may be technique, or it may signal a need for increased development of wrist and forearm muscle groups. Many training devices are available to strengthen grip and forearm muscles, although a simple alternative is to regularly squeeze a rubber ball. You can also adapt certain training devices to simulate the golf swing. For example, a resisted swing can be practiced by attaching an old club to a Mini Gym, Exergenie, Apollo, or pulley weights.

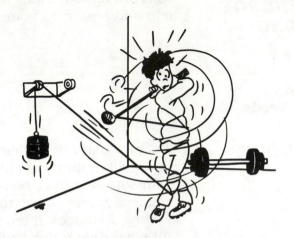

Energy Fitness

Energy fitness demands are low but some endurance is needed to maintain a high level of skill performance throughout a long match or tournament. Based on an analysis of the energy needs in golf, the following energy training methods were listed in Table 6.5.

- Continuous slow running
- Hills
- Hiking carrying a backpack (additional sport-specific training method not included in Table 6.5)

During the off-season, have your golfers maintain their aerobic fitness with easy-paced exercise. Hill striding carrying a weighted pack is an effective sport-specific training method. Consider also hiking or backpacking as off-season activities in addition to the more traditional forms of exercise such as running, cycling, and swimming.

Designing a Training Program

The recommendations for muscular and energy fitness for golfers have been integrated into a sample seasonal plan, illustrated in Table 8.4.

Based on this sample program, you should be able to develop more specific programs to suit your individual athletes. Try to keep your sessions varied but still follow the general training principles outlined. Golfers do have fitness needs that must be met, but even more important is skill improvement. If you coach one of the other highly technical sports like archery or shooting, your fitness program should follow a similar pattern of development.

Table 8.4
Sample Seasonal Training Program for Golf

	Off-Season	Preseason	Competitive Seasons

Muscular fitness	Training emphasis: Strength (3x/week)
	1. Weight training
	  • half squat
	  • arm curl
	  • military press
	  • bent-knee sit-ups
	  • wrist curl
	  • incline press
	  • upright rowing
		Training emphasis: Power (3x/week)
		1. Weight training
		  • apply power-training principles
		  • vary exercises to add variety
		2. Circuit training with weights and calisthenics
		3. Use isokinetic devices to develop power (e.g., resisted golf swing)
		4. Regular flexibility exercises, especially for lower back and shoulders
			Training emphasis: Skills, maintaining muscular fitness
			1. Muscular fitness maintenance program as necessary (1 to 2x/week max)

Energy fitness	Training emphasis: Aerobic foundation (2x/week) 1. Continuous running 2. Hiking, backpacking 3. Rowing, cycling, swimming for recreation	Training emphasis: Maintain aerobic fitness (2 to 3x/week)	Training emphasis: Maintaining aerobic fitness (1x/week) 1. Use continuous exercise as relaxation following intense competition
Skills	Learn and practice new golf techniques	1. Refine and practice skills	1. Concentrate on skill improvement 2. Regular competition 3. Use competitive drills that simulate competition intensity

SAMPLE PROGRAM FOR MEDIUM-MUSCULAR, LOW-ENERGY TRAINING: BASEBALL

This sample program is for baseball, another high-skill sport. In the past, many highly skilled professionals were able to get by with a minimum of off-season training, but that is changing. Today players at all levels engage in muscular and energy training to improve performance and to minimize the risk of injury.

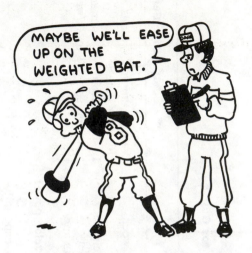

Identifying Fitness Needs

Muscular Fitness

Muscular fitness demands for baseball are higher than for golf. Power is probably the most important component, so strength, speed, and power training should be emphasized in the muscle groups used in running, throwing, and hitting. Muscles of the upper body are especially important in baseball. For pitchers and catchers, muscular endurance is a necessary quality. And all players need to maintain flexibility. From Table 4.3 the following muscle groups and exercises were identified as beneficial for baseball:

Muscle Groups	Weight-Training Exercises
Lower and upper back, upper legs	Half squat
Upper leg	Knee (leg) extension
Upper leg	Leg curl
Lower leg	Heel raise
Chest	Bench press
Chest	Bent-arm pullover
Chest	Straight-arm pullover
Upper arm	Incline press
Upper and lower arm	Arm curl
Shoulder, upper arms	Military press
Shoulder, upper arms	Triceps extension
Shoulder	Upright rowing
Abdomen	Bent-knee sit-ups (with twist)
Trunk, shoulder girdle	Power clean
Trunk, shoulder girdle	Swing with weighted bat
Forearm	Wrist curl or wrist roller
Forearm	Reverse wrist curl

From this list you must select 8 to 10 exercises that best meet the needs of your own ball players. If isokinetic training devices are available, use these to develop power in upper body muscle groups. Many of these devices can be adapted to permit simulation of baseball hitting and throwing actions. Just as for golf, try to think of ways to add resistance to throwing and swinging motions.

Energy Fitness

Baseball is primarily an anaerobic activity. Plays involve intense effort for a duration of no more than a few seconds. However, because baseball games can last several hours and require the ability to recover quickly following intense activity, players should possess an adequate aerobic foundation. In Table 6.5 the following energy training methods were identified for baseball:

- Continuous exercise—slow and fast
- Short anaerobic intervals
- Sprints
- Starts
- Shuttle runs

Clearly, baseball is a game of fast reactions and quick stop-and-go movements. The type of endurance developed by long-distance running is inappropriate for baseball players. During the off-season easy-paced, continuous running or fartlek is ideal for maintaining aerobic fitness and for controlling weight. It also prepares players for the more intense exercise that must follow. A modification to the speed training methods noted above is to have athletes perform sprints while you hold them back with a rope attached to a wide belt. Try to make speed work specific to the sport by having players run bases or by practicing infield drills, run downs, cut-offs, or other related plays.

Designing a Training Program

These ideas and suggestions for formulating muscular and energy fitness training programs have been integrated into a general seasonal plan for baseball, shown in Table 8.5.

Use this general plan to develop specific programs suited to the age and ability of your athletes. Depending on your players, you may want to consider individualizing training for specific positions. For your pitchers and catchers, additional strength and power for the legs, arms, and shoulders may be beneficial. If you are not sure how to apply any of these training ideas, refer to the advice given in previous chapters. Remember, also, to add your own ideas, provided they follow the training principles outlined. Coaches of similar sports that have medium-muscular and low-energy demands should use this model to develop programs for their own sports.

Table 8.5
Sample Seasonal Training Program for Baseball

	Off-Season	Preseason	Competitive Seasons
Muscular fitness	Training emphasis: Strength (3x/week) 1. Weight training • half squat • bench press • incline press • triceps extension • bent-knee sit-ups • power clean • wrist roller 2. Isokinetic strength exercises 3. Regular flexibility exercises	Training emphasis: Power (3x/week) 1. Weight training • apply power-training principles • vary exercises to add variety 2. Circuit training with weights and calisthenics 3. Use isokinetic devices to develop power (e.g., resisted throwing and swinging movements) 4. Regular flexibility exercises, especially for lower back and shoulders	Training emphasis: Skills, maintaining muscular fitness 1. Muscular fitness maintenance program as necessary (1 to 2x/week max)
Energy fitness	Training emphasis: Aerobic foundation (2x/week) 1. Continuous running—vary between fast and slow) 2. Fartlek 3. Participate in other recreational activities to maintain aerobic fitness and control weight	Training emphasis: Anaerobic ability (2x/week) 1. Fartlek of increasing intensity to provide transition to speed work 2. Interval training, hollow sprints, sprints, starts, and shuttle runs 3. Sport-specific drills	Training emphasis: Maintaining anaerobic fitness (1x/week) 1. Schedule high-intensity anaerobic maintenance programs several days before competition to permit full recovery 2. During busy competitive schedule eliminate anaerobic sessions 3. Do easy aerobic runs on off or travel days
Skills	1. Learn and practice new, individual techniques	1. Refine/practice individual and team skills 2. Develop/practice playing strategies 3. Introduce practice drills that simulate competition intensity	1. Regular competition 2. Competitive practice drills modeled after game situations 3. Improve team strategy and individual performance deficiencies

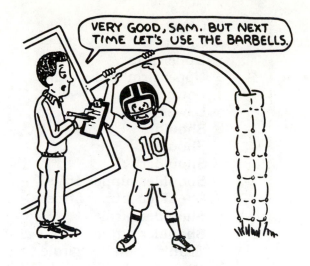

SAMPLE PROGRAM FOR HIGH-MUSCULAR, LOW-ENERGY TRAINING: FOOTBALL LINEMEN

Identifying Fitness Needs

In the last decade almost every major high school and college football program has instituted an extensive off-season weight program. Many colleges have added a strength and conditioning coach to direct these programs. The program included here shows you how to apply basic training principles and methods to improve the fitness of a football lineman or any other athlete in a sport that has high-muscular and low-energy fitness demands.

Muscular Fitness

A high level of muscular fitness is vital for football linemen. The major requirements are for strength and power in the muscle groups used in blocking and tackling. These are total body movements and demand the development of the muscles of the neck, arms and shoulders, and trunk and legs. Each skill has specific needs: Blocking relies on extension strength from the tricep muscle group in the upper arms, while tackling demands flexion strength from the biceps muscle group also in the upper arm. To properly apply the principle of specificity, training should be individualized for offensive and defensive players. All linemen should work to improve speed and to maintain adequate flexibility.

Table 4.3 provides an extensive list of recommended weight-training exercises to develop the muscle groups used by linemen. These are listed below, according to body area.

Muscle Group	*Weight-Training Exercises*
Upper legs	Knee (leg) extension
Upper legs	Leg curls
Lower and upper back, upper legs	Half squat (thigh parallel to floor)

Chest	Bench press
Chest	Bent-arm pullover
Chest	Straight-arm pullover
Upper arm	Incline press
Upper arm and shoulder	Bar dips
Lower back	Back extension
Lower leg	Heel (toe) raise
Shoulder	Press behind neck
Shoulder	Shoulder shrug
Shoulder	Upright rowing
Shoulder, upper arms	Military press
Shoulder, upper arms	Triceps extension
Shoulder girdle	Bent-over rowing
Shoulder girdle	Pulldown-lat machine
Trunk, shoulder girdle	Power clean
Neck	Neck flexion and extension
Abdomen	Bent-knee sit-ups
Upper and lower arm	Arm curl
Forearm	Wrist curl or wrist roller
Forearm	Reverse wrist curl

The length of this list is explained by the variety of skills required in football. For a lineman, you must look more closely at the choices and select the *best* exercises to develop the specific skills linemen need. Remember, however, this will not only depend on the position, but also on each athlete's existing abilities. Coaches must try to identify individual strengths and weaknesses and design training programs based on this knowledge.

In addition to weight training, linemen will benefit from isokinetic training to develop power and from sport-specific training devices such as the leaper and blocking sled. During the preseason, competitive blocking and tackling drills will motivate players as well as improve muscular fitness.

Energy Fitness

Football is an anaerobic sport, played at high speed for a short duration. However, this does not mean you can ignore an adequate aerobic foundation. Players need to be ready for further all-out effort. The major energy-training methods that were listed in Table 6.5 include the following:

- Continuous exercise—slow and fast
- Hills
- Fartlek
- Short anaerobic intervals
- Sprints
- Shuttle runs and starts

Off-season and early preseason training should include some lower intensity exercise such as fast-paced, continuous running and fartlek to prepare the players for the main anaerobic focus to follow. As the competitive season approaches, concentrate almost exclusively on high-intensity anaerobic workouts. Increasing speed of movement over short distances (patterned after game situations) will improve competitive performances.

Designing a Seasonal Training Program

Muscular and energy fitness training recommendations for football linemen have been developed into a seasonal training plan in Table 8.6.

Let me emphasize that this is the starting point for developing a program to meet your athletes' specific fitness needs. Depending on the level of athletes you coach, you may want to increase or decrease training frequency and intensity. But these are minor deviations that can easily be incorporated into your personal seasonal training plan. With some modifications this plan will meet the fitness needs of most football players; it also models a pattern that coaches of other high-muscular, low-energy fitness sports should follow.

SAMPLE PROGRAM FOR MEDIUM-MUSCULAR, MEDIUM-ENERGY TRAINING: BASKETBALL

Most leading basketball players developed their skills during many years of practice on the playground and on the court. But now the game has become so competitive that just playing the game is no longer enough. Muscular and energy fitness training are essential when preparing athletes for peak performances in competition.

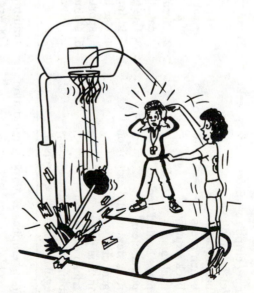

Identifying Fitness Needs

Muscular Fitness

Developing the muscle groups required for jumping, shooting, passing, and rebounding is the key to meeting the muscular fitness needs of basketball players: Arm and shoulder muscle groups are used in shooting, passing, and rebounding; leg muscles are crucial for jumping and running; and

Table 8.6
Sample Seasonal Training Program for Football Linemen

	Off-Season	Preseason	Competitive Seasons
Muscular fitness	Training emphasis: Strength (3x/week) 1. Weight training • half squat[a] • bench press • back extension[b] • heel raise • press behind neck • power clean • neck flexion and extension • arm curl • incline press • tricep extension 2. Isokinetic strength exercises 3. Regular flexibility exercises	Training emphasis: Power, speed (3x/week) 1. Weight training • apply power-training principles • vary exercises to maintain interest and to meet individual deficiencies 2. Circuit training with weights and calisthenics 3. Use isokinetic devices to develop power in important muscle groups 4. Use leaper, blocking sled, and other sport-specific training devices 5. Maintain flexibility	Training emphasis: Maintaining muscular fitness 1. Muscular fitness maintenance program (1 to 2x/week)
Energy fitness	Training emphasis: Aerobic foundation (2x/week) 1. Continuous running (vary between fast and slow) 2. Fartlek (increase intensity toward beginning of preseason) 3. Recreational activities to maintain aerobic fitness and control weight	Training emphasis: Anaerobic ability (2x/week) 1. Interval training, acceleration sprints, hollow sprints, sprints, starts, and shuttle runs 2. Hill or step running for variety	Training emphasis: Maintaining anaerobic fitness (1 to 2x/week) 1. Schedule high-intensity anaerobic sessions several days before competition to permit full recovery 2. Do easy aerobic run on off day
Skills	1. Technique improvement	1. Refine/practice individual and team skills and strategies 2. Use drills that simulate competition intensity	1. Regular competition 2. Competitive drills modeled after game situations but with limited contact to avoid injuries 3. Improve team strategy and eliminate individual performance deficiencies

[a]Squats should be done to a level where the bottom of the thigh is parallel to the ground.
[b]This exercise can also be done with players holding weights for additional resistance.

almost any muscle group can be called to action during intense rebounding battles. Strength, endurance, power, and speed are all vital physical qualities. The variety of skills needed to excel in basketball requires all-round physical development. This is evident in the selection of weight-training exercises illustrated earlier in Table 4.3 and now listed below.

Muscle Group	*Weight-Training Exercises*
Upper legs	Leg curls
Upper legs	Knee (leg) extension
Lower and upper back, upper legs	Half squat
Chest	Bench press
Chest	Bent-arm pullover
Lower leg	Heel (toe) raise
Shoulder	Lateral arm raise
Shoulder	Upright rowing
Shoulder girdle	Pulldown-lat machine
Shoulder, upper arms	Military press
Shoulder, upper arms	Triceps extension
Trunk, shoulder girdle	Power clean
Upper and lower arm	Arm curl
Abdomen	Bent-knee sit-ups
Forearm	Wrist curl or wrist roller
Forearm	Reverse wrist curl
Forearm, fingers	Fingertip push-ups

From this wide selection of exercises, select 8 to 10 and organize them into a program for your athletes. Critically examine each exercise as it is described in Appendix A, and ask yourself which exercises best suit your athletes. Because jumping ability is so important in basketball, you may want to consider using isokinetic devices or plyometrics to develop power. An ideal way to combine all these exercises is to design a training circuit.

Energy Fitness

Basketball is typical of those sports that demand constant movement, broken up by short, intense periods of action. Basketball players need a strong aerobic foundation to enable them to sustain continuous motion and to recover quickly from more intense bursts of activity. However, the primary training emphasis must be on developing the anaerobic systems that fuel the body during the critical game plays. From Table 6.5 we can identify the following training methods as being suited for basketball:

- Continuous exercise—slow and fast
- Hills
- Fartlek
- Repetitions

- Short aerobic intervals
- Medium and short anaerobic intervals
- Shuttles

To build a strong aerobic foundation in the off-season, use continuous running and fartlek, increasing exercise intensity into the preseason, thereby readying athletes for speed work. Stadium steps and other natural hills can add variety to these sessions. By the end of the preseason, concentrate on improving anaerobic fitness through running activities and sport-specific competitive drills.

Designing a Seasonal Plan

In Table 8.7 you can see how these recommendations for improving your basketball players' muscular and energy fitness have been integrated into a seasonal training program.

Depending on the skill and experience of your athletes, you may want to introduce slight training modifications to meet the specific fitness needs required in different playing positions. For example, you may want to focus on improving the jumping ability of your guards and the speed of your forwards. Careful exercise selection will achieve these goals. Individualizing the training program is especially important in basketball if you have youngsters who are tall but lack sufficient muscular development. Coaches of other sports with medium-muscular and medium-energy fitness demands can use this basketball program to model training sessions suited to the sport they coach.

SAMPLE PROGRAM FOR HIGH-MUSCULAR, MEDIUM-ENERGY TRAINING: WRESTLING

The best way to achieve the high level of muscular fitness required in wrestling is to engage in the sport itself. But athletes can prepare for participation by doing well-chosen strength, power, and endurance training prior to the season.

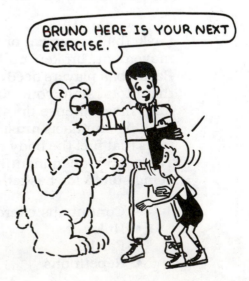

Table 8.7

Sample Seasonal Training Program for Basketball

	Off-Season	Preseason	Competitive Seasons

Muscular fitness	Training emphasis: Strength (3x/week)
	1. Weight training
	  • leg curl
	  • bent-arm pullover
	  • heel raise
	  • pulldown
	  • arm curl
	  • wrist roller
	  • half squat
	  • bench press
	2. Isokinetic strength exercises
	3. Regular flexibility exercises
		Training emphasis: Power, endurance (3x/week)
		1. Weight training
		  • apply power and endurance training principles
		  • vary exercises to add variety
		2. Circuit training with weights and calisthenics
		3. Use isokinetic devices to develop power (e.g., resisted ball pulldown)
		4. Use leaper machine
		5. Plyometrics
		6. Regular flexibility exercises
			Training emphasis: Speed, power (1 to 2x/week)
			1. High-intensity muscular fitness maintenance program

Energy fitness	Training emphasis: Aerobic foundation (2x/week) 1. Continuous running (vary between fast and slow) 2. Fartlek 3. Pick-up games 4. Other recreational activities to maintain aerobic fitness	Training emphasis: Anaerobic ability (2x/week) 1. Fartlek (increasing intensity) 2. Interval training 3. Hollow sprints 4. Sprints, starts, and shuttles 5. Hill or step running for variety	Training emphasis: Maintaining anaerobic fitness (1 to 2x/week) 1. Organize high intensity sessions several days before competition to permit full recovery 2. Use competition to substitute for training during busy playing schedule 3. Do easy aerobic run on travel and off days
Skills	1. Learn and practice new individual techniques	1. Refine/practice individual and team skills 2. Develop/practice playing strategies 3. Introduce practice drills that simulate competition intensity	1. Regular competition 2. Competitive practice drills modeled after game situations (e.g., half-court games) 3. Improve team strategy and individual performance deficiencies

Identifying Fitness Needs

Muscular Fitness

Wrestlers must be prepared to sustain a total effort for several minutes; therefore, muscular fitness, especially muscular endurance and power, is critical when training wrestlers. Because wrestling involves the total body, a systematic program must be designed to exercise the upper and lower body muscle groups used for holding, lifting, and throwing opponents. Table 4.3 helps you identify the crucial muscle groups that wrestlers must train and offers the following list of suggested weight training exercises:

Muscle Groups	*Weight-Training Exercises*
Upper legs	Knee (leg) extensions
Lower and upper back, upper legs	Half squat
Chest	Bench press
Upper and lower arm	Arm curl
Lower back	Back extension
Shoulders, upper and lower arm	Parallel bar dip
Shoulder, upper arms	Military press
Shoulder girdle	Pulldown-lat machine
Shoulder girdle	Bent-over rowing
Trunk, shoulder girdle	Power clean
Trunk	Twisting motion with pulley weights
Abdomen	Bent-knee sit-ups
Neck	Neck flexion and extension
Forearm	Reverse wrist curl
Forearm	Wrist curl or wrist roller

Notice how several exercises train similar muscle groups. This choice increases variety and reduces the likelihood of boredom, which often occurs when athletes constantly repeat the same exercise routine. It also permits individualization of the program to suit your athletes' special needs. Clearly, you would want to design different programs if one athlete needs to improve leg strength and another has poor upper body strength.

In addition to these weight training exercises, special training devices, including a Leaper machine or football blocking sled, can benefit your athletes. If isokinetic training devices are available, you should identify exercises to train the specific muscle groups used in wrestling. Additional muscular fitness training ideas, especially for off-season endurance development, might include paddling a canoe or kayak, rowing a boat, swimming, arm-cranking a stationary bicycle, and other continuous upper body exercises.

Energy Fitness

The short duration of wrestling bouts places major demands on the body's anaerobic systems. However, wrestlers do need some aerobic ability to assist fast recovery between bouts and to sustain energy throughout day-long tournaments. Running, cycling, and rowing are ideal training modes. In Table 6.5 the following training methods were recommended for wrestlers:

- Continuous exercise—slow and fast
- Hills
- Short aerobic intervals
- Medium and short anaerobic intervals

To prepare your athletes for these intense sessions, use the off-season and early preseason to develop a solid aerobic foundation. Fartlek and continuous exercise is ideal preparation. Remember, however, that the primary focus must be on the anaerobic energy pathways, so concentrate on this for most of the preseason and throughout the competitive seasons.

Designing a Seasonal Training Program

In Table 8.8 the recommendations for muscular and energy fitness training are integrated into a sample seasonal training program for wrestling.

This advice provides you with a starting point to develop your own program. You now need to develop specific programs suited to your athletes' abilities that can be practically implemented. Using the advice given in the previous chapters, you should be able to determine suitable levels of exercise intensity. Also, you are probably aware of many more training ideas used in wrestling that apply the basic principles outlined. By applying these general principles and by adding ideas gleaned from other coaches or previous experience, you will have all the essential ingredients for a successful program. Coaches of similar sports that have high-muscular and medium-energy fitness requirements should pattern their training programs after the wrestling model.

SAMPLE PROGRAM FOR MEDIUM-MUSCULAR, HIGH-ENERGY TRAINING: SWIMMING (400 FREESTYLE AND ABOVE)

Swimming is a good example of a high-energy sport. Like running, cross-country skiing, and other endurance sports, swimming requires many hours of energy training each week. Young swimmers seem capable of regularly performing hard endurance workouts. Perhaps because the water is a forgiving medium, swimmers usually remain free from the nagging injuries that plague runners when they increase their mileage.

Table 8.8

Sample Seasonal Training Program for Wrestling

	Off-Season	Preseason	Competitive Seasons
Muscular fitness	Training emphasis: Strength (3x/week) 1. Weight training • knee extension • half squat • bench press • arm curl • back extension • parallel bar dip • pulldown-lat machine • bent-knee sit-ups 2. Isokinetic strength exercises	Training emphasis: Power, endurance (3x/week) 1. Weight training • vary exercises to add variety • vary sessions to apply power and endurance training principles 2. Circuit training with weights and calisthenics 3. Use isokinetic devices to develop power 4. Use leaper, blocking sled, or other training devices 5. Maintain flexibility	Training emphasis: Speed, power (1 to 2x/week) 1. Muscular fitness maintenance program 2. Sport-specific power and speed drills that simulate competition intensity
Energy fitness	Training emphasis: Aerobic foundation (2x/week) 1. Fartlek 2. Continuous running (vary between fast and slow 3. Rowing, cycling, and swimming for recreation	Training emphasis: Anaerobic ability (2x/week) 1. Fartlek (increasing intensity) 2. Interval training, acceleration sprints, hollow sprints, sprints, starts, and shuttle runs 3. Hill or step running for variety	Training emphasis: Maintaining anaerobic fitness (1 to 2x/week) 1. Organize high-intensity sessions several days before competition to permit full recovery 2. Competition may substitute for training during busy schedule 3. Do easy aerobic runs on off or travel days
Skills	1. Learn and practice new skills	1. Refine/practice skills 2. Integrate energy training into sport-specific drills	1. Regular competition 2. Competitive drills that simulate competition intensity

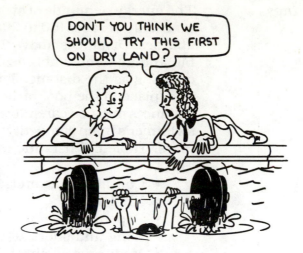

Identifying Fitness Needs

Muscular Fitness

Swimmers need strength to pull themselves through the water, endurance to keep it going, and power and speed to perform at competitive speed. Arm, shoulder, and back muscles must be given the primary training emphasis. From Table 4.3 we can identify the following muscle groups needing development as well as the recommended weight training exercises.

Muscle Groups	Weight-Training Exercises
Lower and upper back, upper legs	Half squat
Chest	Bench press
Chest	Bent-arm pullover
Lower back	Back extension
Shoulder	Upright rowing
Shoulder girdle	Bent-over rowing
Shoulder, upper arms	Military press
Shoulder, upper arms	Triceps extension
Shoulder, upper and lower arm	Parallel bar dip
Trunk	Leg raise
Trunk	Bent-knee sit-up

In addition to a selection of these weight training exercises, many swim coaches have invented special training methods specifically for swimmers. Using elastic bands, pulleys, Biokinetic, Exergenie, Mini-gym, and other devices based on the isokinetic principle, swimmers can model typical arm actions of all the swimming strokes. And as for wrestlers, off-season activities that exercise the upper body, such as canoeing, rowing, or kayaking, are ideal for swimmers.

Energy Fitness

The energy demands of swimming depend on the racing distance. Short races (50 to 200 m) require speed and anaerobic abilities. Distances above 200 m demand a mixture of aerobic and anaerobic abilities, with the aerobic proportion increasing as the distance lengthens. Energy training should take place in the pool rather than on the running track, and distances must be carefully selected to be consistent with each swimmer's main competitive event. For 400-m freestyle swimmers, Table 6.5 lists the following training methods:

- Continuous exercise—slow and fast
- Fartlek
- Repetitions
- Long and short aerobic intervals
- Medium and short anaerobic intervals
- Sprints
- Starts

At this distance, endurance or aerobic ability is crucial for good performances. However, as you will notice, most of the swimming should be at a fairly high pace. During the off-season, easy-paced swimming to help maintain a minimal level of aerobic fitness is fine, but this training is not specific enough to have much effect on improving competitive performances. Over 400 m, top swimmers are working at the upper end of their aerobic capacity and are depending on a raised anaerobic threshold to support intense racing efforts.

Another limitation of slow swimming is that because the stroke is not performed at close to competitive speed, the muscle groups are not rehearsing the same action required of them during a race. This point is worth stressing to all coaches: Practicing a skill at a speed different from that required in competition ignores the key training principle of *specificity*.

Designing a Seasonal Training Program

Muscular and energy fitness recommendations for training a 400-m freestyler have been integrated into a seasonal program in Table 8.9.

A difference between swimming and the other sports that have been considered is that energy fitness training for swimming simultaneously practices the same skills needed during competition. The same is true for other sports such as running, cycling, rowing, and skiing where skills are developed during energy fitness training. Improvements occur simultaneously in both areas. This explains why two to five energy fitness training sessions may be held each week.

Swimming coaches face the challenge of juggling frequency and intensity to ensure that both *skill* and *fitness* improve at the appropriate rates. Without careful design, a training program could improve an athlete's fitness but fail to rectify

Table 8.9

Sample Seasonal Training Program for a 400-m Freestyle Swimmer

	Off-Season	Preseason	Competitive Seasons
Muscular fitness	Training emphasis: Strength (3x/week) 1. Weight training • half squat • bent-arm pullover • back extension • bent-over rowing • triceps extension • leg raise • bench press • parallel bar dip 2. Isokinetic strength exercises 3. Regular flexibility program	Training emphasis: Endurance, power (3x/week) 1. Weight training • apply endurance and power training principles • vary exercises for variety to meet individual needs 2. Special isokinetic or other training devices designed for swimmers 3. Circuit training 4. Regular flexibility program	Training emphasis: Endurance, speed (1 to 2x/week) 1. Muscular fitness maintenance program • adjust according to individual endurance or speed needs
Energy fitness	Training emphasis: Aerobic foundation (2 to 3x/week) 1. Fast, continuous swimming 2. Fartlek (land and in pool) 3. Interval training in pool (moderate intensity) 4. Kayaking, rowing, canoeing for recreation	Training emphasis: Aerobic/anaerobic threshold (3x/week) 1. Fartlek 2. Interval training 3. Repetitions (85% max HR) • Model practices on race distances and/or time. Simulate competition intensity	Training emphasis: Anaerobic threshold (2 to 5x/week) 1. Fartlek 2. Interval training 3. Repetitions • Vary pace to include opportunities for technique emphasis (arms, legs, turns, etc.) plus competition at high-intensity
Skills	1. Learn and practice new techniques	1. Refine/practice techniques	1. Regular competition 2. Competitive drills

a basic skill deficiency. Conversely, a program could improve skills but have no effect on fitness. Coaches of similar sports should take care to distinguish skill development from fitness training. Further skill refinement may be essential for training to have its desired effect.

A particular danger with these types of sports is overtraining, a topic discussed in the next chapter. Training must suit the age and experience of your athletes. Repetitious sports like swimming, running, cycling, skating, and rowing are notorious for boredom and burnout, so keep practices interesting by including a wide variety of games and relays. Regularly include easy days or days off to keep your athletes motivated. Then as the competitive season arrives, ease down on your training schedule. After all, you don't want your athletes to produce their best efforts in the training pool.

As a final note, if you coach young swimmers, avoid encouraging early specialization in one swimming stroke. Youngsters should be proficient in all strokes. If they begin to excel in one stroke as they get older, this may be the time to permit specialization. However, potential talent is often not so easy to identify nor isolate. History is full of cases where average athletes have changed from one stroke to another, or even one sport to another, before realizing their full athletic potential.

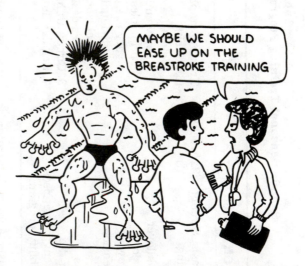

SUMMARY

1. This chapter illustrated how to apply the theories and principles of sport physiology in practice.

2. All coaches need to develop fitness programs based on the muscular and energy fitness needs of their sport and the differing physical characteristics of their individual athletes.

3. Seasonal training variations must be considered. Four training phases can be distinguished, each of which de-

mands a different training emphasis; these include the off-season, preseason, early season, and peak season.

4. The process of developing seasonal training programs for several sports was explained so that coaches would feel competent to design appropriate programs for their own athletes.

PART 5
Performance

Chapter 9
Peak Performances

Peak performances, personal records, and lifetime bests seldom occur by chance. More often than not they are the product of careful preparation. The competitive peak is the culmination of a well-planned training program. This final chapter introduces some additional topics that can significantly affect your athletes' performances.

SETTING TRAINING GOALS

Improvements in muscular and energy fitness take time. Setting training goals can be an effective way of sustaining your athletes' interest toward fitness training. Ideally, coaches and athletes should set these goals together, agreeing on a reasonable rate of expected improvement. The key to goal setting is always to remain *realistic*. If athletes constantly face goals that are unobtainable, instead of stimulating greater effort, athletes become discouraged and quickly lose interest.

Goals must also be relevant to your sport. For long-distance runners, goals set in time or training miles per week might be appropriate. For linebackers, increases in strength measured in pounds or repetitions are probably more relevant. Consider the type of realistic training goals that would appeal to your athletes; then work with each individual to establish a rate of progress that is challenging but achievable. Goal setting is discussed in greater detail in the *Coaches Guide to Sport Psychology* (Martens, in press).

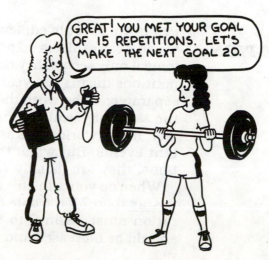

GREAT! YOU MET YOUR GOAL OF 15 REPETITIONS. LET'S MAKE THE NEXT GOAL 20.

KEEPING RECORDS

Because training goals are achieved slowly, athletes should be encouraged to keep daily records of progress toward seasonal training goals. These records can be either simple notes indicating daily mileage or detailed accounts of the day's program and/or of progress figures, including strength or endurance improvements, changes in body weight, and resting and exercise pulse rates.

Psychologists emphasize the value of record keeping to increase feedback and motivation. Appropriate feedback reinforces desired behaviors: Encouraging athletes to keep training records will increase their motivation to train regularly. Highly motivated athletes will also be better prepared to overcome obstacles that hinder the training of less interested athletes. For example, if one of your athletes has to leave town for a week, will the training schedule still be followed? That schedule is more likely to be followed if a training log stares the athlete in the face every day! Success in sport—and in life, for that matter—goes to persistent, determined, unrelenting individuals who have goals and constantly work hard toward them.

As well as helping your athletes set weekly, monthly, seasonal, and even long-term training goals, you should keep a written record of their progress. If injury or illness causes a setback, have them adjust their sights and get back to work; remind them that this happens to everyone. If the goals were reasonable in the first place, they may still be attainable.

COMPETITIVE PEAKS

Everyone is searching for peak experiences—thrills and highs. There is no greater satisfaction in life than doing your best, than playing your best game. Once you have had that feeling, you will never forget it. How do athletes achieve a competitive peak, and once there, stay at that level as long as possible? They begin with proper preparation.

PHYSICAL PREPARATION

Peaks are short-lived; few last more than a month. Even the world's top athletes do not attempt to sustain a peak for very long; it only seems they do. Instead, they pick out several competitions during the year and attempt to peak for each one, separately. In between they continue to compete, but not with the same physical and mental preparation and intensity. In fact, many world class athletes occasionally lose less important events. But when the time comes for the big competitions, they are usually ready to excel.

When do your athletes need to peak? How long do they hope to stay there? If the date is May 15, their final physical preparation must begin 6 to 8 weeks before. Training intensity should be increased and early competitions used to sharpen their performance. Tell your athletes to think less about winning and more about quality of effort. Have them sharpen their form and work on speed. Make sure they reduce training volume, get plenty of rest, and eat sensibly, especially as the important date approaches. Finally, athletes should always keep track of their body weight and use the last few weeks to achieve their best competitive weight.

The Taper Period

Seven to 14 days before the event, athletes must further reduce their training. Gradually reduce the quantity or volume of training to allow complete recovery. Many athletes have achieved personal records after a minor injury forced a period of rest. The taper period allows the athletes to recover from the demands of regular training and minor injuries and increases athletes' motivation to compete. Intelligent coaches build toward the peak season and use the taper to be sure their athletes are healthy enough to enjoy it.

Schedule only easy stretching and form work in the days immediately preceding a competition. Have athletes avoid any drugs in the last few days, including aspirin and antihistamines. Tell them to avoid stimulants like coffee or tea the night before a competition so they can get a normal night's sleep. (They should not try to get more or less sleep than they are used to.) If they are too excited to fall asleep, they should not fret; they are still getting needed rest.

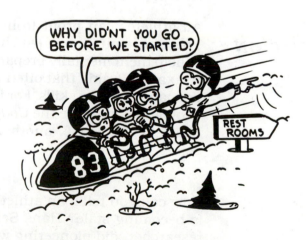

Competition Day

If the athletes intend to eat before competition, be sure they allow at least 3 hours between eating and the event. Remind them to warm up adequately and to check the weather conditions, their equipment, and any other factors that could affect performance. Do their shoes need laces? blisters need treatment? ankles need taping? Do they need special medication? Do not let your athletes neglect anything of importance (even that all-important last minute trip to the bathroom).

It is a good idea for each athlete to go through a checklist with a friend or teammate to make sure he or she has *everything* needed for the competition. This technique may prevent your athletes from repeating the experience Mike had on competition day. Mike trained for months to get ready for a 50-km cross-country ski marathon. When race day came, he got up early, ate a good breakfast, took care of personal matters, and set about preparing his skis for the race. He carefully warmed glide wax into the ski tip and tail, heated a tough binder into the kick zone, and followed this with four thin coats of wax, a necessary precaution for a long race. When everything seemed ready, he went to the starting line to test the wax and to warm up. Seconds before the starting gun, as the announcer emphasized the importance of wearing the correct race number, Mike realized that his racing bib was back at the motel. As he dashed across the street to get the number, he heard the starter's gun. Minutes later, he set out in pursuit of the pack, a frustrated but wiser skier.

In some events, athletes must be prepared for unexpected changes, for example, the weather. Skiers need extra wax when the temperature changes. Runners and bikers must be prepared for rain, wind, or snow. Many football teams have lost because they were not equipped with the correct shoes for an icy field. Coaches must try to think of everything their athletes might need, including extra food, water, clothing, or equipment.

MENTAL PREPARATION

All athletes can profit from improved mental preparation. There are a number of psychological skills athletes can learn to help them mentally prepare for competition. These include relaxation (a skill that often needs to be learned), concentration, and imagery skills. For information on how to teach psychological skills, see the *Coaches Guide to Sport Psychology* (Martens, in press), another volume in the ACEP Level 2 series.

The Stress of Training

How can you tell if an athlete is overtraining, or if he or she is becoming stale? Hans Selye (1956), a famous Canadian researcher, did pioneering work on the subject of stress. He found that a number of stressors, such as infections, emotional disturbance, or extreme exertion or exhaustion, could significantly impair physical performance. If the stressors were severe enough or if they persisted, the body's resistance would break down, often with harmful side-effects. Thus, it is important for all coaches to be aware of the signs and symptoms of staleness, overtraining, and stress.

Staleness

The term *staleness* implies something is getting old, or deteriorating. When sport ceases to be fun or when other factors conspire to dampen your athletes' interest, staleness often develops. Listed below are some common symptoms and causes of staleness.

Common Symptoms and Causes of Staleness

SYMPTOMS	CAUSES
Chronic fatigue	Lack of rest/sleep
Irritability	Unchanging routine
Decreased interest	Emotional problems
Weight loss	Overwork/study
Reduced speed, strength, endurance	Poor diet
Slower reflexes	Overtraining
Poor performance in sport, school, or work	

Several factors can cause staleness. An inadequate diet can produce staleness in several ways. For example, one young miler found his running times consistently falling off throughout the season. When he finally realized that his vegetarian experiment could be the cause and returned to a sound diet, his performance began to improve. He discovered the hard way that special diets require special knowledge. Poor eating habits can also produce hypoglycemia or low blood sugar. Symptoms of hypoglycemia include nervousness, fatigue, irritability, dizziness, and confusion. Simple changes in diet can clear up these problems and get athletes back on the right track. Refer to the *Coaches Guide to Nutrition and Weight Control* (Eisenman & Johnson, 1982) for more information on diet.

Other physical sources of staleness are low-grade infections such as colds, bronchitis, flu, or undetected allergies. Psychological sources sometimes include personal problems, being involved in too many activities, or having an unusually large load at school or at work. All these factors can interrupt your athletes' ability to concentrate and can drain both their emotional and physical energy.

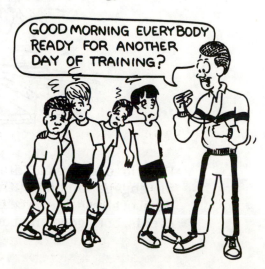

Overtraining

To ensure your athletes experience steady progress, be alert to the signs of overtraining. Simple measures such as resting pulse, body weight, and oral temperature can indicate overtraining or impending infection. Enforced rest at the appropriate time can save hours of lost practice time. Other obvious signs, such as minor injuries, may signal impending exhaustion. Encourage your athletes to listen to their bodies and to accept what they hear. They should not practice if they feel too tired, and if they do not feel ready for a long, hard workout, give them an easier alternative. Six overtraining indices that athletes can use to track their physiological condition are listed in Table 9.1. Have your athletes try the indices for a couple of weeks; then select those indices that seem to be most useful. This is another area in which good coach-athlete communication is critical. Listen to your athletes, and do not risk their health by trying to force them past their immediate physiological limitations.

Physiologists are currently experimenting with more sophisticated indicators of overtraining: White blood cell counts indicate infection; hemoglobin or other blood measures show fatigue; lactic acid levels show the intensity of a workout; certain enzymes in the blood indicate muscle breakdown; and hormone levels indicate excess stress. Although these and other measures may be available to competitors on the Olympic team, they are neither available nor essential for most athletes. The body has a way of telling you when to rest. As long as your athletes listen to their bodies and you listen to your athletes, many problems can be avoided.

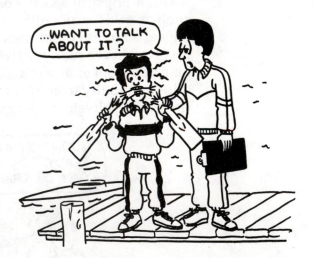

Stress

Emotional stress can drain enthusiasm and sap energy. People engage in competitive athletics because they enjoy the thrill of stress, but excessive stress can be harmful. Many life events, both good and bad, contribute to a stress buildup. Too

Table 9.1
Overtraining Indices

Index	Evaluation
Pulse	Take your pulse rate daily (for 60 s) in the morning before you arise. Average the daily rates. When the morning pulse is 5 or more beats above the average, you should suspect overtraining or illness.
Temperature	Take your morning temperature daily for a week to establish your "normal," then use it whenever the morning pulse is elevated. A fever usually indicates infection. Take the day off.
Weight	Take your weight daily, in the morning (after toilet but before breakfast). Average daily weights. A rapid or persistent weight loss could indicate impending problems due to poor eating habits, failure to replace fluids, nervousness, or excessive fatigue.
Fluid	At the end of the day, rate your fluid intake. Failure to replace fluids could lead to dehydration exhaustion. 5—much above average 4—above average 3—average 2—below average 1—much below average
Sleep	Every morning for a week, rate the quality of your sleep; consider ease of falling asleep. A persistent drop in quality or quantity calls for a rest. 5—much above average 4—above average 3—average 2—below average 1—much below average
Fatigue	In the morning after you arise, rate your tiredness. Persistent fatigue calls for a rest. 1—ready to drop 2—extremely tired 3—very tired 4—slightly tired 5—about average 6—somewhat fresh 7—very fresh 8—extremely fresh 9—full of life

much at one time can lead to burnout. Common causes of stress include the following:

- a death in the family
- major illness or injury
- divorce of parents

- financial problems
- trouble at school
- trouble with the law

Less obvious events, even happy ones, can contribute to stress buildup, for example:

- holiday
- vacation
- change in social or recreational habits
- change in residence or school
- personal achievement

In addition, athletes are often exposed to stressful situations as the following:

- travel, including time zone changes
- sleep loss
- exhaustive competition or practice
- personal factors, relationships, living conditions

Coaches must be alert to these stressors and not hesitate to make adjustments when necessary. Often a minor change is all that is needed to reduce the stress. If an athlete is overworked, prescribe a rest; if athletes are bored during a long vacation, introduce a new work or training routine; if the pressure of the sport becomes excessive, suggest a diversion or release.

Coaches have a responsibility to help their athletes resolve stressful situations; help them to analyze the situation, list possible solutions, then select and attempt remedies. If it appears the demands of work, school, family, friends, and sport are pulling in too many directions, help the athlete decide which ones are most important (at this time) and fit them into a schedule. Encourage young athletes to talk to their teachers, family, friends, and fellow athletes and to explain why they cannot work as much or play as much as they would like.

More information on techniques for controlling stress is available in the *Coaches Guide to Time Management* (Kozoll, 1985) and the *Coaches Guide to Sport Psychology* (Martens, in press).

SUMMARY

1. Peak performances are generally the product of careful preparation.

2. Athletes should set training goals to guide and to motivate their efforts and should keep a written record of their achievements.

3. Training programs should be planned so that your athletes peak for important competitions.

4. On competition days a checklist will help athletes and coaches remember crucial details.

5. Psychological skills training can improve mental preparation.

6. Excessive stress can impede peak performances. To avoid the negative consequences of stress, coaches and athletes should remain alert for the symptoms of staleness, overtraining, and distress.

CONCLUSION

Earlier in the book you were introduced to the principle of moderation. Moderation applies to all aspects of life. Dedication is fine as long as it is tempered by judgment and moderation. Too much of anything can be bad for both physical and psychological health. Train too hard, too fast, or too long and the body begins to deteriorate. Encourage your young athletes to practice moderation in all things. Do *not* let them sacrifice long-term goals to achieve immediate success. Allow them to approach training with moderation, knowing that overtraining is far more disastrous than undertraining. Success comes to those who pace themselves. Some burn brightly and then fade; others are in the race until the end, practicing good judgment, self-discipline, and above all, moderation.

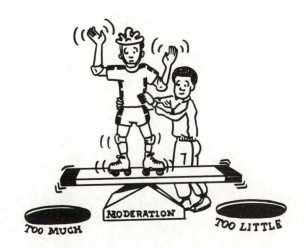

Appendix A
Flexibility Exercises

Bent-Knee Stretch   *Muscles:* Lower back and hamstrings

Directions:

1. Grasp ankles and pull until you feel the stretch.
2. Hold five counts and relax. Repeat.

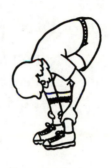

Toe Pull   *Muscles:* Groin and thighs

Directions:

1. Pull on toes while pressing legs down with elbows.

Variation: Lean forward and try to touch head to feet or floor.

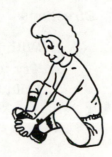

Seated Toe Touch   *Muscles:* Back and hamstrings

Directions:

1. With toes pointed, slide hands down legs until you feel stretch.
2. Hold five counts and relax.
3. Now grasp ankles and pull until head approaches legs, then relax.
4. Draw toes back and slowly attempt to touch toes with your hands.

Variation: Try with legs apart.

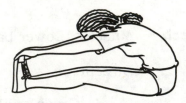

Leg Pull   *Muscles:* Hamstrings and gluteal (rear) muscles

Directions:

1. Pull leg toward and across chest.
2. Feel stretch high in hamstring.
3. Hold five counts and relax.

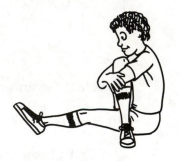

Backover   *Muscles:* Hamstrings and low back

Directions:

1. With knees bent bring legs over head.
2. Try to touch floor with toes until you feel stretch.
3. Hold for five counts, then relax.

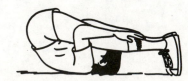

Stride Stretch

Muscles: Inside thigh muscles (groin)

Directions:

1. Assume stride position with hands on floor or chair for balance.
2. Feel stretch, hold, then relax.
3. Put arm and shoulder inside front leg to accentuate stretch.

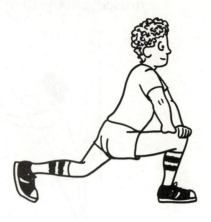

Side Stretch

Muscles: Arms and trunk

Directions:

1. Grasp hands above head and slowly bend to one side.
2. Push gently, hold and relax.
3. Switch sides.

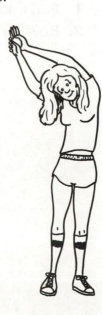

Wall Stretch

Muscles: Calves and Achilles tendon

Directions:

1. Stand about 3 ft from wall, feet slightly apart.
2. Lean forward, keep heels on floor, and feel stretch in calves.

Variation: Concentrate on one leg at a time. Contract calf muscle briefly, then relax and feel stretch in Achilles tendon.

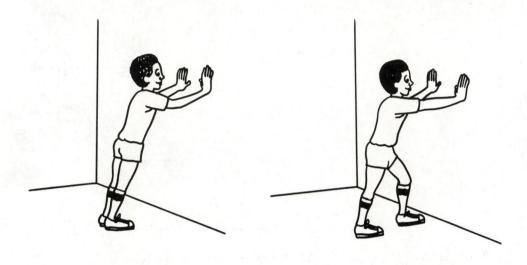

Shoulder Stretch

Muscles: Shoulders

Directions:

1. Pull arms back until partner feels stretch.
2. Hold for five counts, then relax.

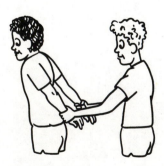

**Back and Leg
Stretch**

Muscles: Lower back, hamstrings, and gluteal muscles

Directions:

1. Pull ankles to feel stretch.

Variation: With practice try to touch fingers or palms to the floor.

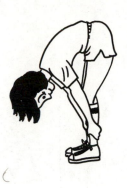

The Bow

Muscles: Arms, back, legs

Directions:

1. Bow at waist.
2. Put hands on wall and feel stretch from hands to heels.

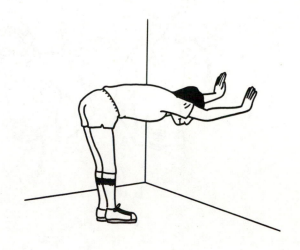

Side Twist

Muscles: Trunk and lower back

Directions:

    1. With arms extended to side, twist as far as possible.

    2. Hold, then twist back and repeat.

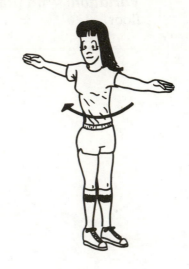

Neck Circles

Muscles: Neck, shoulders, and upper back

Directions:

    1. Gently roll head in full circle, first to one side, then the other.

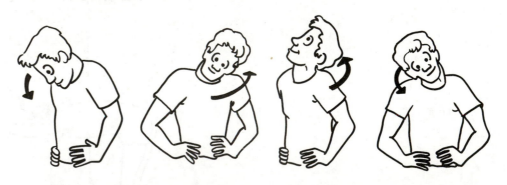

The Hug   *Muscles:* Shoulders and upper back

Directions:

1. Hug yourself as tightly as possible.
2. Hold, relax, and repeat.

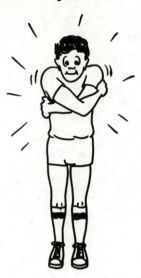

Try to think up additional flexibility exercises suited to your sport. Follow the same exercise techniques described above and in chapter 4.

Appendix B
Weight Training and Resistance Exercises

These exercises are arranged alphabetically for easy referencing. If you wish to exercise a specific body part, refer to Table 4.3 for recommended exercises.

Arm Curls

Muscles: Arm flexors (biceps)

Directions:

1. Either sit or stand.
2. Grasp the bar with an underhand grip.
3. Flex arms to lift bar up to shoulders.
4. Use only the arms to perform this movement, do *not* permit the body to swing. (This is easier to control if the athlete performs the exercise in a sitting position.)

Variation: Same exercise can be performed with a reverse or overhand grip.

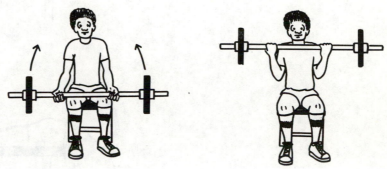

Arm Curls cont.

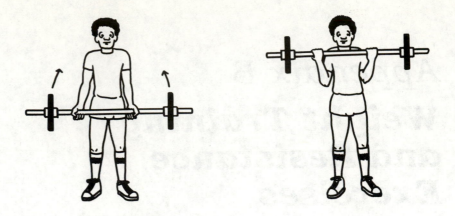

Back Extension

Muscles: Lower back

Directions:

1. Use a bench that supports the hips and allows feet to be fixed. (This can be achieved by having a partner hold athlete's lower legs down.)

2. Lock fingers behind head and bend so that head is close to floor.

3. Lift upper body as high as possible, then slowly lower and repeat.

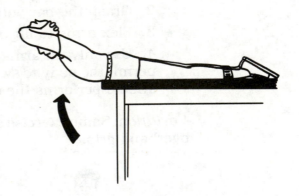

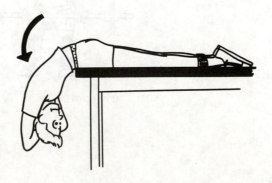

Bench Press

Muscles: Chest, shoulders, and arms

Directions:

1. Hands hold bar a little wider than shoulder width apart.

2. Spotter(s) helps position bar above shoulders.

3. Bar is lowered to chest, then pushed back above shoulders.

4. Keep feet, hips, and head down on bench while exercising.

5. Spotter(s) helps return bar when exercise is completed.

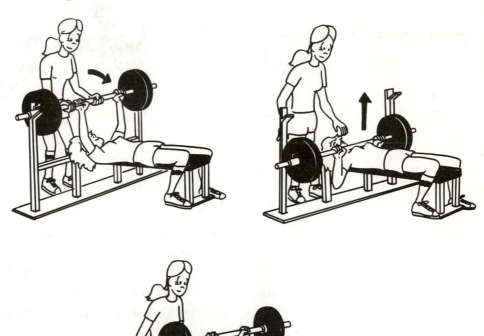

Bent-Arm Pullover

Muscles: Chest, shoulder and arm extensors

Directions:

1. Lay on bench with head and upper shoulders supported.

2. Reach back to bar placed on floor close to bench.

3. Use overhand grip with hands close together.

4. Lift weight over head and lower down onto chest.

5. Try to keep elbows tucked in near to head throughout movement.

Variation: Use dumbbells instead of bar.

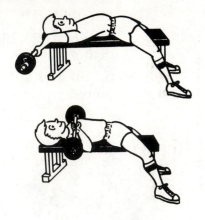

Bent-Knee Sit-Ups   *Muscles:* Abdomen

Directions:

1. Sit with knees bent, hands crossed over chest, and chin tucked in.

2. Begin sit-up by first lifting the head, then shoulders, then the remaining upper body parts.

3. Lift until elbows touch knees, then lower body back to floor.

Variations:

1. Sit-ups can also be performed with feet fixed.

2. Exercise difficulty can be increased by sitting athlete on an inclined bench or by holding a weight close to chest throughout the exercise.

Note. Sit-ups should *not* be performed with straight legs.

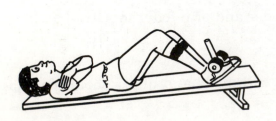
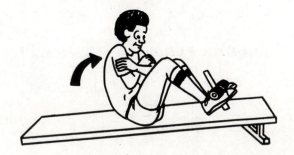

Bent-Over Rowing   *Muscles:* Shoulder girdle

Directions:

1. Hold bar with overhand grip, hands slightly more than shoulder-width apart.
2. Feet apart, bend at waist so that trunk is almost parallel to the floor, head in line with trunk.
3. Slightly bend knees to relieve tension on lower back.
4. Pull bar directly to chest, lower, and repeat.

Variations:

1. Can be done with dumbbells.
2. Pull bar to different parts of chest.
3. Placing head on a waist-high head support will help prevent trunk movement and will relieve stress on lower back.

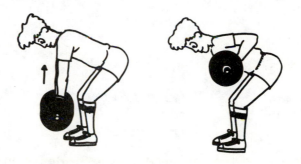

Half Squat   *Muscles:* Lower and upper back, upper legs

Directions:

1. *Always* wear a weight belt and have *two* spotters available to lift and support weight when using free weights.
2. Bar is placed on a rack just below shoulder height.
3. Athlete steps under bar, positions feet slightly wider than shoulder width with feet pointing outward.
4. Keep heels flat, back straight, and head up (focusing on a mark on the ceiling may help).
5. Lift weight off rack, bend knees to lower weight until thighs are parallel with floor.
6. Straighten knees, using leg and hip muscles to lift weight.
7. Keep *back straight* and *head up* throughout the lift.

Variation:

1. Use leaper machine (isokinetic).

Note. Use light weights until movement has been thoroughly learned. Do *not* bend knees lower than parallel with floor position.

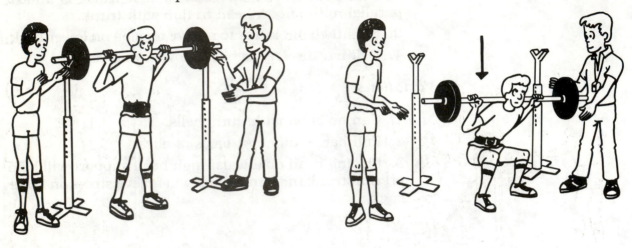

Heel Raises

Muscles: Lower leg

Directions:

1. Stand under pads of calf machine with ball of foot on a block and the heel suspended.
2. Keep knees locked and lift heels as high as possible.
3. Lower to permit heels to drop below block.

Note. This exercise can be performed on a calf machine, leg press machine, or with free weights. When using free weights, the athlete can hold a heavy weight close to thighs or balanced on shoulders.

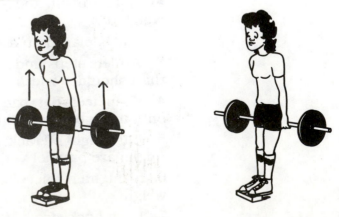

Incline Press

Muscles: Upper chest, shoulders, and arms.

Directions:

1. Athlete sits on 45° inclined bench and grips bar with hands shoulder width apart.

2. Use spotters to help lift weight into position (can begin exercise in either up or down position).

3. Push bar directly upwards, keeping elbows tucked in tight to the body.

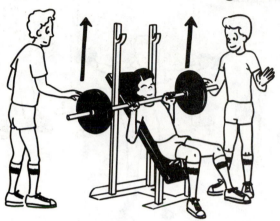
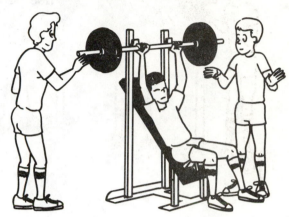

Knee Extension

Muscles: Upper leg (quadriceps)

Directions:

1. Use leg extension machine.

2. Place both feet under the padded bars and lift smoothly.

3. Hold bench with hands or cross hands in front of chest.

4. Keep lift smooth and do *not* use swinging movement with upper body to assist.

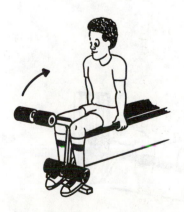
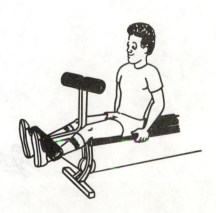

Lateral Arm Raise

Muscles: Shoulder

Directions:

1. Hold dumbbells with palms facing inward, feet slightly apart.
2. Raise weights level to head, keeping knuckles on top.
3. Hold momentarily, then lower and repeat.
4. Exercise can be done sitting to eliminate tendency to use body to lift weights.

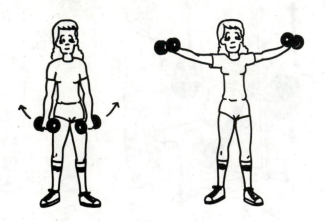

Leg Curl

Muscles: Upper legs (hamstrings)

Directions:

1. Lay on stomach on leg curl machine.
2. Extend legs fully under lifting bar of machine.
3. Flex legs as far as possible.
4. Lower weight and repeat.

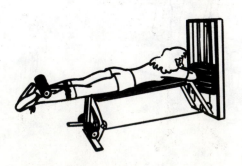 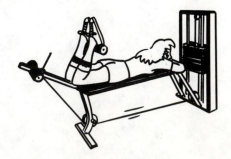

Leg Raise

Muscles: Trunk

Directions:

1. Hold wall bar or overhead bar with palms facing outward.
2. Lift legs until they are parallel to ground.
3. Lower legs and repeat.

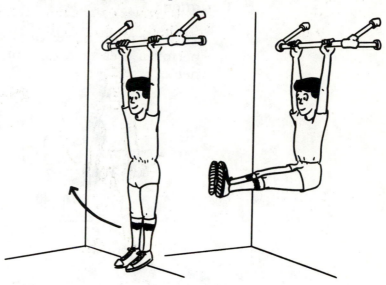

Military Press

Muscles: Shoulders, upper chest, and back

Directions:

1. Grip bar with hands shoulder width apart.
2. Rest bar on chest approximately level with collar bone to begin.
3. Push bar straight upward using arms and shoulder muscles.
4. Keep back straight.

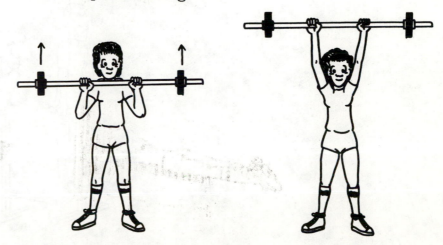

**Neck Flexion
and Extension**

Muscles: Neck

Directions:

1. Movements are performed using a neck harness.
2. Athlete sits with hands on thighs holding body firm.
3. Weight is lifted and lowered.

Variation:

1. Many of the newer variable resistance training devices permit a greater variety of exercises to strengthen the neck.

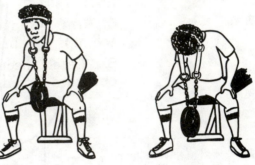

Parallel Bar Dip

Muscles: Shoulder, upper and lower arm

Directions:

1. Support the body with straight arms
2. Lower the body until the chest is level with the bars.
3. Explosive push to lift body to starting position.

Variation:

1. Suspend weights from a waist belt to increase resistance.

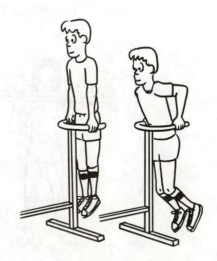

Power Clean

Muscles: Trunk, shoulder girdle, and legs

Directions:

1. Athletes should *always* wear a weight belt when performing this exercise.

2. Bar is grasped with an overhand grip about shoulder width apart.

3. Back and arms are straight, hips low, and eyes focused ahead.

4. Lift begins with drive from the legs and hips, arms remaining straight, and bar kept close to the athlete's body.

5. Arms begin to bend as the body is fully extended and the hips are thrust forward.

6. "Catch" occurs as the knees quickly bend and the elbows are forced forward under the bar.

7. The feet hop slightly forward between the extension and catch.

8. The bar is lowered first to the thigh-support position, then to the floor.

Note: This is an advanced lift and *not* recommended for young or beginning athletes.

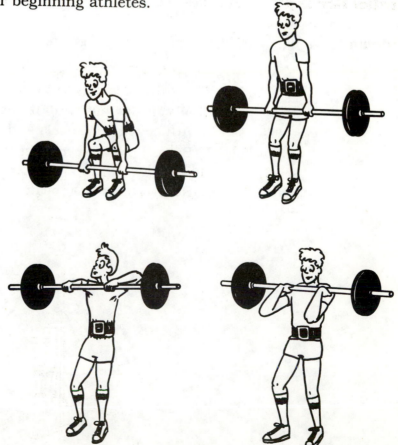

Press Behind Neck   *Muscles:* Shoulders and arm extensors (triceps)

Directions:

1. Grip bar with hands shoulder width apart.
2. Rest bar on shoulders to begin with feet slightly apart.
3. Push bar straight upward using arms and shoulder muscles.
4. Keep back straight.

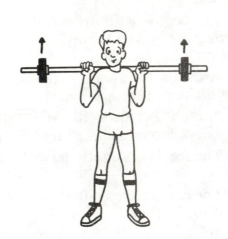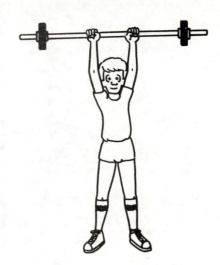

Pulldown   *Muscles:* Lower and upper back

Directions:

1. Must use some form of a lat machine.
2. Athlete sits or kneels and holds bar with wide grip.
3. Bar is pulled down *behind* the back until it touches the shoulders.
4. Return bar and repeat.

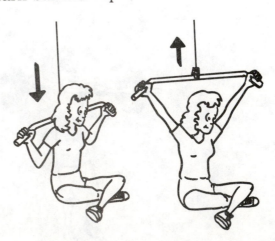

Reverse Curl

Muscles: Wrist extensors and elbow flexors

Directions:

1. Either sit or stand.
2. Grasp the bar with an overhand grip.
3. Flex arms to lift bar up to shoulders.
4. Use only the arms to perform this movement; do *not* permit the body to swing. (This is easier to control if the athlete performs the exercise from a sitting position.)

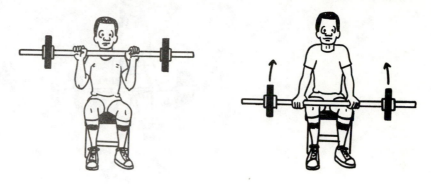

Reverse Wrist Curl

Muscles: Wrist extensors

Directions:

1. Hold bar with overhand grip, hands about shoulder width apart.
2. Athlete sits and forearms rest on thighs.
3. Keeping forearms fixed, allow weight to fully extend wrists, then flex wrists to lift weight as far as possible forward.

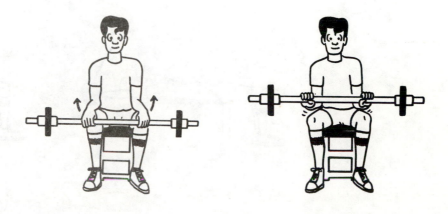

Shoulder Shrug   *Muscles:* Shoulder girdle

Directions:

1. Use overhand grip with hands approximately shoulder width apart.
2. Hold weight at thigh level and shrug shoulders pulling them as close to ears as possible.
3. Keep arms straight throughout entire movement.

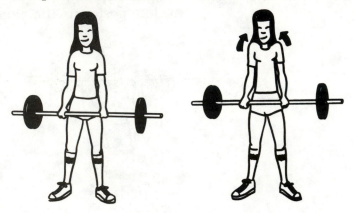

Straight Arm Pullover   *Muscles:* Chest, shoulder, and upper arm extensors

Directions:

1. Lay on bench with head and upper shoulders supported.
2. Use overhand grip with hands shoulder width apart.
3. Hold weight over chest with arms straight.
4. Slowly lower bar until arms are parallel with floor, then lift through the same arc to starting position.

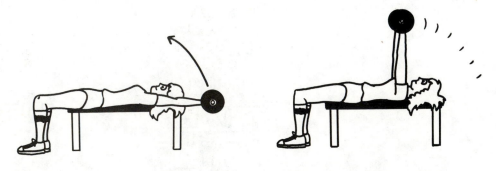

Triceps Extension   *Muscles:* Shoulder and upper arm (especially arm extensors)

Directions:

1. Use overhand grip with hands close together.
2. Hold weight directly above head with arms fully extended.
3. Lower weight behind head, keeping elbows close to head.
4. Lift weight to starting position and repeat.

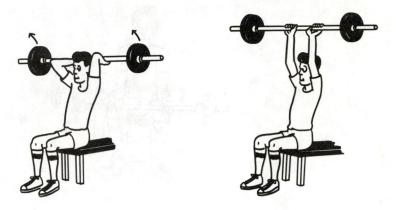

Upright Rowing   *Muscles:* Shoulder and arm flexors

Directions:

1. Use overhand grip with hands close together.
2. Pull the bar to the chin, keeping the elbows above the bar.
3. Lower weight to thigh level and repeat.

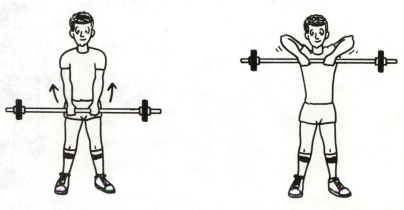

Wrist Curl

Muscles: Wrist flexors

Directions:

1. Hold bar with underhand grip, hands about shoulder width apart.

2. Athlete sits and forearms rest on thighs.

3. Keeping forearms fixed, allow weight to fully extend wrists, then flex wrists to lift weight as far as possible forward.

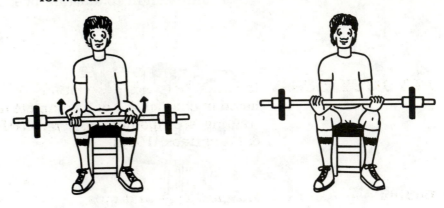

Wrist Roller

Muscles: Wrist flexors

Directions:

1. Use light weight attached by rope to a short wooden bar.

2. Roll wrists to roll rope around bar and lift weight.

3. Unroll rope and repeat.

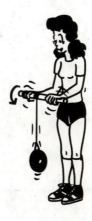

Appendix C
Plyometric Training Exercises

PLYOMETRICS

Included here are descriptions of the plyometric exercises listed in chapter 4. For a complete description of plyometric training, see *Plyometrics: Explosive Power Training* (Radcliffe & Farentinos, 1985).

Double Leg Bound

Muscles: Legs and hips

Directions:

1. Begin in half-squat position with arms at side, back straight, and head up.
2. Jump vigorously forward and upward, throwing arms forward.
3. Try to straighten body in air before landing.
4. Land into half-squat position and repeat.

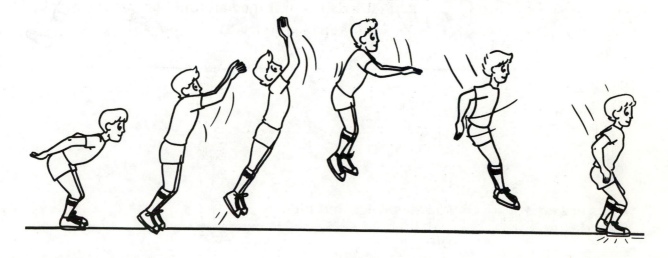

**Alternate Leg
Bound**

Muscles: Legs and hips

Directions:

1. Stand with one foot in front, arms relaxed at sides.
2. Push off with back leg and drive front knee toward chest.
3. Try to jump as far and high as possible before landing.
4. Drive off from other leg after landing.

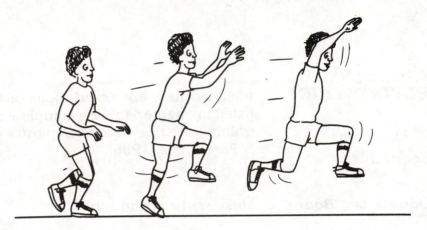

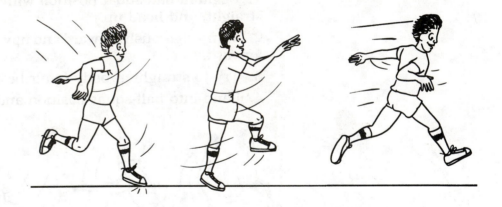

**Double Leg
Speed Hop**

Muscles: Legs and hips

Directions:

1. Stand with back straight, head up, and shoulders slightly forward.
2. Arms should be bent to about 90°.

3. Jump upward as high as possible, bringing knees up to chest and using arms for lift.

4. On each landing, try to take off quickly.

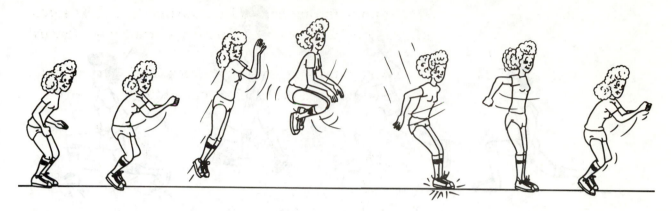

Squat Jump

Muscles: Hips, thighs, and lower leg

Directions:

1. Stand upright with feet about shoulder width apart.

2. Lock fingers and hold palms against back of head.

3. Begin by dropping quickly to half-squat position, checking this motion and exploding upward as high as possible.

4. Repeat movement immediately on landing.

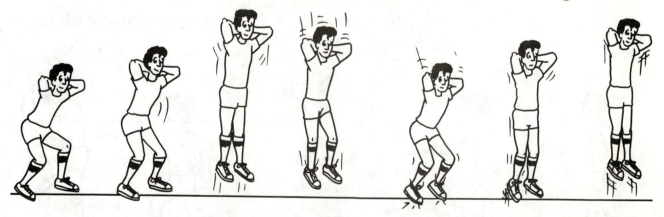

Split Jump

Muscles: Lower back, thighs, hips, and lower leg

Directions:

1. Stand with one leg forward, the other just behind midline of body.

2. Jump up as high and straight as possible, using the arms to get extra height.

3. Absorb landing shock by bending forward knee and spring upward again.

4. Repeat exercise with other leg in forward position.

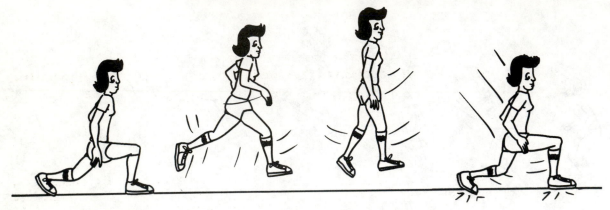

Skipping

Muscles: Hips, rear, thigh, and lower leg

Directions:

1. Stand relaxed with one leg forward.
2. Drive off back leg for short skipping step.
3. Thrust knee to chest and lift with arms.
4. Try to "hang" in the air.
5. Land and repeat using other leg.
6. Movement pattern should be *right-right-step-left-left-step*, and so on.

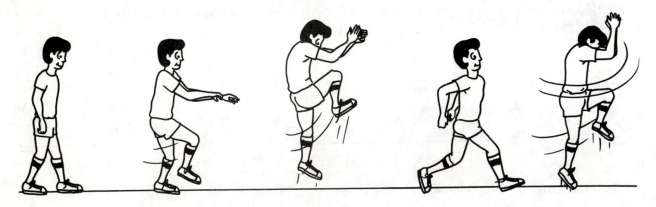

Medicine Ball Twist/Toss

Muscles: Abdominals, back, hips, arms, and chest

Directions:

1. Cradle ball next to body at waist height.
2. Twist quickly in opposite direction to intended throw.
3. Abruptly check this motion by twisting quickly in direction of intended throw and releasing ball to partner.
4. Concentrate on using hips as well as arms to throw the ball.

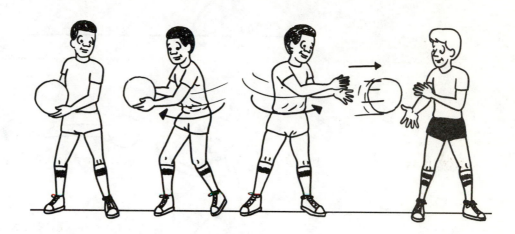

Medicine Ball Chest Pass

Muscles: Chest, upper back, shoulders, wrist, and forearm

Directions:

1. Choose medicine ball your athletes can handle.
2. Stand or sit facing a partner.
3. Hold ball at chest, hands a little behind ball and arms bent.
4. Partner anticipates throw by extending arms toward thrower.

5. Push ball forcefully to partner who catches by breaking the ball's momentum then immediately pushes ball back in opposite direction.

6. Passes continue back and forth.

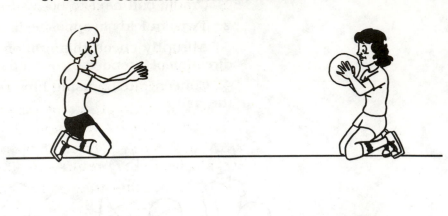

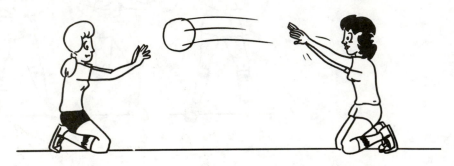

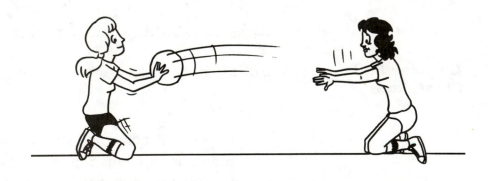

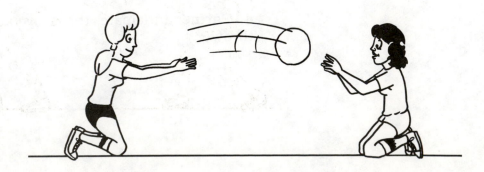

Heavy Bag Thrust   *Muscles:* Arms, chest, shoulders, back, and hip

Directions:

1. Use heavy punching bag suspended on rope.
2. Face bag with legs split; foot next to bag is back.
3. Put inside hand on bag at chest height, fingers pointing upward.
4. Keep elbow close to body and arm bent.
5. Use body to push bag away forcefully, fully extending arm to follow through.
6. Catch return of bag with open hand, and push forward again *before* bag returns to starting position.
7. Change sides to exercise other side of body.

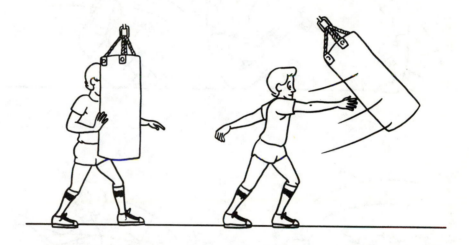

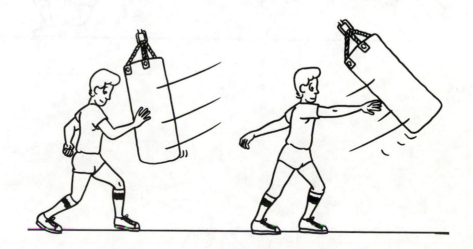

Floor Kip

Muscles: Hips, abdominals, lower back, shoulders, arms, and thighs.

Directions:

1. Sit with legs together and feet pointed.
2. Keep legs extended and knees together and roll backward.
3. Place hands with palms down, on either side of head.
4. Quickly extend legs upward and forward while pushing with hands.
5. Bend legs to land in semi-squat position.

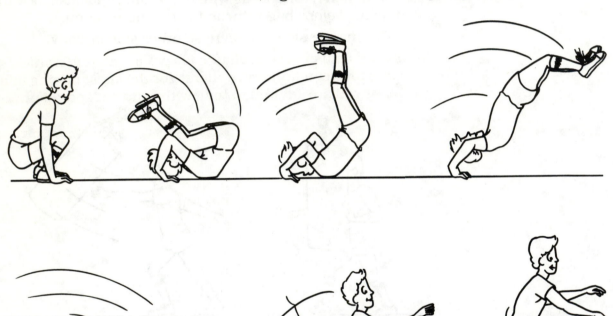

Appendix D
Information for Purchasing Skinfold Calipers

Skinfold calipers are available for prices ranging from a few dollars to over a hundred dollars. For the latest pricing information you are advised to review the current sport journals. Some of the available products and the addresses and phone numbers of their manufacturers are listed below (in descending order of cost):

Product: Lange Skinfold Calipers
Address: Cambridge Scientific Industries
P.O. Box 265
Cambridge, MD 21613
Phone: (301) 376-3124

Product: Lafayette Skinfold Calipers
Address: Lafayette Instrument Co.
P.O. Box 5729
Sagamore Parkway
Lafayette, IN 47903
Phone: (800) 428-7545
(317) 423-1505

Product: Slimguide Calipers
Address: Creative Health Products, Inc.
882 Saddle Ridge Rd.
Plymouth, MI 48170
Phone: (800) 742-4478
(312) 453-5309

Product: Fat-O-Meter
Fat Control Caliper
Address: American Alliance Publications
Sales Unit
1900 Association Drive
Reston, VA 22091
Phone: (703) 476-3481

Product: Fat-O-Meter
Address: Novel Products
80 Fairbanks, Unit 12
Addison, IL 60101
Phone: (312) 628-1787

Product: Adipometer Skinfold Caliper
Address: Ross Laboratories
Attn. Educational Services
625 Cleveland Ave.
Columbus, OH 43216
Phone: (614) 227-3333

References

Astrand, P.O., & Rodahl, K. (1977). *Textbook of work physiology: Physio-logical bases of exercise*. New York: McGraw-Hill.

Balke, B. (1963). *A simple field test for the assessment of physical fitness*. (Report No. 63-6). Oklahoma City: Civic Aeronautic Research Institute, Federal Aviation Agency.

Cooper, K.H. (1970). *The new aerobics*. New York: Bantam.

Eisenman, P., & Johnson, D.A. (1982). *Coaches guide to nutrition and weight control*. Champaign, IL: Human Kinetics.

Fox, E.L. (1984). *Sport physiology*. Philadelphia, PA: Saunders College Publishing.

Frederick, E. (1973). *The running body*. Mountain View, CA: World Publications.

Kozoll, C. (1985). *Coaches guide to time management*. Champaign, IL: Human Kinetics.

Martens, R. (in press). *Coaches guide to sport psychology*. Champaign, IL: Human Kinetics.

Martens, R., Christina, R.W., Harvey, J.S., Jr., & Sharkey, B.J. (1981). *Coaching young athletes*. Champaign, IL: Human Kinetics.

Radcliffe, J.C., & Farentinos, R.C. (1985). *Plyometrics: Explosive power training* (3rd ed.). Champaign, IL: Human Kinetics.

Runner's World. (1973). *Runner's training guide*. Mountain View, CA: World Publications.

Selye, H. (1956). *The stress of life*. New York: McGraw-Hill.

Sharkey, B.J. (1974). *Physiological fitness and weight control*. Missoula, MT: Mountain Press.

Sharkey, B.J. (1975). *Physiology and physical activity*. New York: Harper & Row.

Sharkey, B.J. (1977). *Fitness and work capacity*. Washington, DC: U.S. Government Printing Office.

Skinner, J., & McLellan, T. (1980). The transition from aerobic to anaero-bic metabolism. *Research Quarterly for Exercise and Sport*, **51**, 234-248.

Wilt, F. (1968). Training for competitive running. In H.B. Falls (Ed.), *Exercise physiology* (pp. 395-414). New York: Academic Press.

Glossary of Physiological Terms

Acclimatization—Adaptation to an environmental condition such as heat or altitude.

Accommodating resistance—Resistance adjusts to meet the changing force capabilities of the contracting muscle as in isokinetic (same speed) contractions.

Actin—Muscle protein that works with the protein myosin to produce movement.

Adipose tissue—Tissue in which fat is stored.

Aerobic—In the presence of oxygen; aerobic metabolism utilizes oxygen.

Aerobic capacity—Maximal oxygen intake in liters per minute.

Aerobic fitness—Maximum ability to take in, transport, and utilize oxygen.

Aerobic power—Maximal oxygen intake in milliters per kilogram of body weight per minute (ml/kg/min).

Agility—Ability to change direction quickly while maintaining control of the body.

Alveoli—Tiny air sacs in the lungs where O_2 and CO_2 exchange takes place.

Amino acids—Form proteins; different arrangements of the 22 amino acids form the various proteins (muscles, enzymes, hormones, etc.).

Anaerobic—In the absence of oxygen; nonoxidation metabolism.

Anaerobic threshold—When aerobic metabolism no longer supplies all the need for energy, energy is produced anaerobically; indicated by increase in lactic acid.

ATP—Adenosine Triphosphate—high-energy compound formed from oxidation of fat and carbohydrate. Used as energy supply for muscle and other body functions; the energy currency.

Atrophy—Loss of size of muscle; when muscle isn't used, it doesn't turn to fat, it atrophies.

Balance—Ability to maintain equilibrium while in motion.

Blood pressure—Force exerted against the walls of arteries.

Bronchiole—Small branch of airway; sometimes undergoes spasm, making breathing difficult, as in exercise-induced bronchospasm (EIB).

Buffer—Substance in blood that soaks up hydrogen ions to minimize changes in acid-base balance (pH).

Calories—Amount of heat required to raise 1 kilogram of water 1° centigrade (same as kilocalorie).

Capillaries—Smallest blood vessels (between arterioles and venules) where oxygen, foods, and hormones are delivered to tissues and carbon dioxide and wastes are picked up.

Carbohydrate—Simple (sugar) and complex (potatoes, rice, beans, corn, grains) foodstuff used for energy; stored in liver and muscle as glycogen—excess is stored as fat.

Carbohydrate loading (glycogen loading)—A procedure that elevates muscle glycogen stores.

Cardiac—Pertaining to the heart.

Cardiac output—Volume of blood pumped by the heart each minute; product of heart rate and stroke volume.

Cardiorespiratory endurance—Synonymous with aerobic fitness or maximal oxygen intake.

Cardiovascular system—Heart and blood vessels.

Central nervous system (CNS)—The brain and spinal cord.

Cholesterol—Fatty substance formed in nerves and other tissues. Excessive amounts in blood have been associated with increased risk of heart disease.

Concentric contraction—Shortening of the muscle during contraction.

Constant resistance—Resistance doesn't change, as in weight lifting.

Contraction—Development of tension by muscle: *concentric*—muscle shortens; *eccentric*—muscle is lengthened under tension; *static*—contraction without change in length.

Coronary arteries—Blood vessels that originate from the aorta and branch out to supply oxygen and fuels to the heart muscle.

Counterforce—Resistance exercises with a partner to provide isokinetic contractions in a technique physical therapists call proprioceptive neuromuscular facilitation.

Creatine phosphate (CP)—Energy-rich compound that backs up ATP in providing energy for muscles.

Dehydration—Loss of essential body fluids.

Diastolic pressure—Lowest pressure exerted by blood in artery; occurs during resting phase (diastole) of heart cycle.

Eccentric contraction—Lengthening of the contracted muscle, as when lowering a heavy weight.

Elastic recoil—Release of elastic energy in a muscular contraction brought about by a brief stretch or preload.

Electrocardiogram (ECG)—A graphic recording of the electrical activity of the heart.

Electrolyte—Solution of ions (sodium, potassium) that conducts electric current.

Electromyogram (EMG)—A recording of the electrical activity that immediately precedes muscular contractions to determine the degree of muscular involvement.

Endurance—The ability to persist, to resist fatigue.

Energy balance—Balance of caloric intake and expenditure.

Enzyme—An organic catalyst that accelerates the rate of chemical reactions.

Epinephrine (adrenalin)—Hormone from the adrenal medulla and nerve endings of the sympathetic nervous system; secreted during times of stress to help mobilize energy.

Evaporation—Elimination of body heat when sweat vaporizes on surface of skin. Evaporation of 1 liter of sweat yields a heat loss of 580 calories.

Exercise—Sometimes applied specifically to calisthenics; usually denotes any form of physical activity—synonymous with effort, exertion, physical activity, etc.

Fartlek—Swedish term meaning speed play; a form of training where participants vary speed according to mood as they run through the countryside.

Fast glycolytic fiber (FG)—Fast-twitch muscle fiber with limited oxidative capability; easily fatigued.

Fast oxidative glycolytic fiber (FOG)—Fast-twitch fiber with oxidative and glycolytic capabilities.

Fat—Important energy source; stored for future use when excess fat, carbohydrate, or protein is ingested.

Fatigue—Diminished work capacity, usually short of true physiological limits. Real limits in short intense exercise due to factors within muscle (muscle, pH, calcium), long-duration effort—glycogen depletion, or CNS fatigue due to low blood sugar.

Flexibility—Range of motion through which the limbs or body parts are able to move.

Glucose—Energy source transported in blood; essential energy source for brain and nervous tissue.

Glycogen—Storage form of glucose, found in liver and muscles.

Heart rate—Frequency of contraction, often inferred from pulse rate (expansion of artery resulting from beat of heart).

Heat stress—Temperature/humidity combinations that lead to heat disorders such as heat cramps, heat exhaustion, or heat stroke.

Hemoglobin—Iron-containing compound in red blood cell that forms loose association with oxygen.

Hypoglycemia—Low blood sugar (glucose).

Inhibition—Opposite of excitation in the nervous system.

Insulin—Pancreatic hormone responsible for getting blood sugar into cells.

Interval training—Training method that alternates short bouts of intense effort with periods of active rest.

Ischemia—Lack of blood to specific area like heart muscle.

Isokinetic—Contraction against resistance that is varied to maintain high tension throughout range of motion while speed remains constant.

Isometric—Contraction against immovable object (static contraction).

Isotonic—Contraction against a constant resistance.

Lactic acid—By-product of anaerobic glycolysis.

Lean body weight—Body weight minus fat weight.

Maximal oxygen intake (uptake, consumption)—Aerobic fitness. Best single measure of fitness with implications for health; synonymous with cardiorespiratory endurance (VO_2max).

Metabolism—Energy production and utilization processes, often mediated by enzymatic pathways.

Mitochondria—Tiny organelles within cells; site of all oxidative energy production.

Motoneuron—Nerve that transmits impulse to muscle fibers.

Motor area—Portion of cerebral cortex that controls movement.

Motor unit—Motor nerve and the muscle fibers it innervates.

Muscle fiber types—Fast-twitch fibers are fast contracting but fast to fatigue; slow-twitch fibers contract somewhat slower but are fatigue resistant.

Muscle soreness—Discomfort after exercise.

Muscular fitness—The strength, muscular endurance, and flexibility you need to carry out daily tasks and avoid injury.

Myofibril—Contractile threads of muscle composed of the proteins actin and myosin.

Myoglobin—A hemoglobin-like compound in muscle; helps bind oxygen.

Myosin—Muscle protein that works with actin to produce movement.

Neuron—Nerve cell that conducts impulse; the basic unit of the nervous system.

Obesity—Excessive body fat (over 20% for men, over 30% for women).

Overload—A greater load than normally experienced; used to coax a training effect from the body.

Oxygen debt—Recovery oxygen uptake above resting requirements to replace deficit incurred during exercise.

Oxygen deficit—Lack of oxygen in early moments of exercise.

Oxygen intake—Oxygen used in oxidative metabolism.

Perceived exertion—Subjective estimate of exercise difficulty.

Peripheral nervous system—Parts of the nervous system not including the brain and spinal cord.

Power—The rate of doing work $\frac{(\text{force} \times \text{distance})}{\text{time}}$.

Preload—See Elastic recoil.

Progressive resistance—Training program in which the resistance is increased as the muscles gain in strength.

Protein—Organic compound formed from amino acids; forms muscle tissue, hormones, enzymes, etc.

Pulse—Wave that travels down the artery after each contraction of the heart.

Respiration—Intake of oxygen from atmosphere into lungs and then via the blood to the tissues and exhale of carbon dioxide from tissues to the atmosphere.

Repetition maximum (RM)—The maximum number of times you can lift a given weight (1 RM is the most you can lift one time).

Sarcomere—The contractile unit of the muscle.

Slow-twitch fiber—See Muscle fiber types.

Somatotype—Body types: Ectomorph is linear or thin, mesomorph is muscular, and endomorph is fat.

Speed of movement—Comprised of reaction time—time from stimulus to start of movement, and movement time—time to complete the movement.

Strength—Ability of muscle to exert force.

Stroke volume—Volume of blood pumped from ventricle during each contraction of heart.

Synapse—Junction between neurons.

Systolic pressure—Highest pressure in arteries that results from contraction (systole) of heart.

Tendon—Tough connective tissue that connects muscle to bone.

Testosterone—Male hormone.

Threshold—The minimal level required to elicit a response.

Tonus—Muscle firmness in absence of a voluntary contraction.

Triglycerides—A fat consisting of three fatty acids and glycerol.

Valsalva maneuver—Increased pressure in abdominal and thoracic cavities caused by breath holding and extreme effort.

Variable resistance—Resistance varies as muscle moves through range of motion, as with devices that use cams or oval-shaped pulleys.

Velocity—Rate of movement or speed ($\frac{distance}{time}$).

Ventilation—The amount of air moving in and out of the lungs per minute, the product of respiratory frequency (f) and tidal volume (TV).

Ventricle—Chamber of heart that pumps blood to lungs (right ventricle) or to rest of body (left ventricle).

Weight training—Progressive resistance exercise using weight for resistance.

Wind chill—Cooling effect of temperature and wind.

Work—Product of force and distance.

Index